Diagnostic and Surgical Arthroscopy of the Temporomandibular Joint

Bruce Sanders, DDS

Adjunct Professor
Section of Oral and Maxillofacial Surgery
University of California School of Dentistry
Los Angeles, California
Senior Staff, Saint John's Hospital and Health Center
Santa Monica, California

Ken-Ichiro Murakami, DDS, DMSc

Assistant Professor
Department of Oral and Maxillofacial Surgery
Faculty of Medicine
Kyoto University
Kyoto, Japan

Glenn T. Clark, DDS, MS

Acting Director
Dental Research Institute
Professor and Co-Director
TMJ and Facial Pain Clinic
UCLA Center for the Medical Sciences
Los Angeles, California

1989
W.B. SAUNDERS COMPANY
Harcourt Brace Jovanovich, Inc.

Philadelphia   London   Toronto
Montreal   Sydney   Tokyo

W. B. SAUNDERS COMPANY
Harcourt Brace Jovanovich, Inc.

The Curtis Center
Independence Square West
Philadelphia, PA 19106

Library of Congress Cataloging-in-Publication Data

Diagnostic and surgical arthroscopy of the temporomandibular joint
[edited by] Bruce Sanders, Ken-Ichiro Murakami, Glenn T. Clark.

    p.   cm.
    Includes index.
    ISBN 0-7216-2453-7

    1. Temporomandibular joint—Diseases—Diagnosis.
2.Temporomandibular joint—Surgery. 3. Arthroscopy. I. Sanders,
Bruce, 1943- . II. Murakami, Ken-Ichiro. III. Clark, Glenn T.
[DNLM: 1. Arthroscopy—methods. 2. Temporomandibular Joint-
surgery. 3. Temporomandibular Joint Diseases—diagnosis. WU 140

D536]

RD526.D53   1989   617'.522059—dc19   DNLM/DLC

for Library of Congress   88-26489
                                                    CIP

Editor: John Dyson
Developmental Editor: Linda Mills
Designer: Liz Schweber
Production Manager: Bob Butler
Manuscript Editor: W. B. Saunders Staff
Illustration Coordinator: Walt Verbitski
Page Layout Artist: Liz Schweber
Indexer: Susan Thomas

Diagnostic and Surgical Arthroscopy of the
Temporomandibular Joint   ISBN 0–7216–2453–7

Last digit is the print number: 9   8   7   6   5   4   3   2   1

Dr. Sanders dedicates this book to his wife, Barbara.

Dr. Murakami dedicates this book to his wife, Toshiko.

Dr. Clark dedicates this book to his wife, Nan.

Contributors

FERNANDO BALDIOCEDA, M.S., D.D.S.
Research Associate, UCLA School of Dentistry, Section of Gnathology
and Occlusion, Los Angeles, California
Comparative Imaging Study

CAROL A. BIBB, Ph.D., D.D.S.
Adjunct Assistant Professor, UCLA School of Dentistry, Section of
Gnathology and Occlusion, Los Angeles, California
Comparative Imaging Study

RALPH D. BUONCRISTIANI, D.D.S.
Lecturer, Section of Oral and Maxillofacial Surgery, and Clinical
Instructor, Continuing Education in Dentistry, UCLA School of
Dentistry, Los Angeles, California; Staff Surgeon, St. John's Hospital
and Health Center and Santa Monica Medical Center, Santa Monica,
California; Staff Surgeon, UCLA Medical Center, Los Angeles,
California
*Operating Room Environment; Arthroscopic Technique; Surgical
Arthroscopy*

GLENN T. CLARK M.S., D.D.S.
Professor and Acting Director, UCLA Dental Research Institute, Los
Angeles, California
Analysis of Arthroscopically Treated TMJ Derangement and Locking

M. FRANKLIN DOLWICK, D.M.D., Ph.D.
Professor and Chairman, Department of Oral and Maxillofacial
Surgery, University of Florida, Gainesville, Florida
Introduction

KEVIN M. EHRHART, M.D.
Clinical Instructor, Division of Orthopaedic Surgery, UCLA School of
Medicine, Los Angeles, California; Senior Staff, St. John's Hospital and
Health Center, Santa Monica, California; Senior Staff, Santa Monica
Medical Center, Santa Monica, California; Attending and Faculty,
UCLA Center for Health Sciences, Los Angeles, California
Orthopedic Arthroscopy

DAVID G. MOODY, D.D.S.
Lecturer, Section of Gnathology and Occlusion, UCLA School of
Dentistry, Los Angeles, California
Analysis of Arthroscopically Treated TMJ Derangement and Locking

KEN-ICHIRO MURAKAMI, D.D.S., Ph.D.
Assistant Professor in the Department of Oral and Maxillofacial
Surgery, Kyoto University Faculty of Medicine, Kyoto, Japan
*Arthroscopic Anatomy; Arthroscopic Technique; Diagnostic
Arthroscopy; Treatment Planning; Comparative Imaging Study*

ANDREW G. PULLINGER, L.D.S., B.D.S., D.D.S., M.Sc.
Associate Professor, Section of Gnathology and Occlusion, UCLA
School of Dentistry, Los Angeles, California
*Comparative Imaging Study; Natural History and Pathologic
Progression of Internal Derangements with Persistent Closed Lock*

JOHN B. ROSS, D.D.S.
Lecturer, Section of Oral Radiology, Section of Gnathology and
Occlusion, UCLA School of Dentistry, Los Angeles, California
Treatment Planning; Comparative Imaging Study

BRUCE SANDERS, D.D.S.
Adjunct Professor, Section of Oral and Maxillofacial Surgery, UCLA
School of Dentistry, Los Angeles, California; Senior Staff, Saint John's
Hospital and Health Center, Santa Monica, California
*Operating Room Environment; Arthroscopic Technique; Surgical
Arthroscopy; Analysis of Arthroscopically Treated TMJ Derangement
and Locking; Treatment Planning*

Preface

In September, 1986, the UCLA Dental Research Institute and the UCLA School of Dentistry sponsored a symposium on Diagnostic and Surgical Arthroscopy of the Temporomandibular Joint. The scientific sessions included orthopedic surgery's experience with arthroscopy of the knee and other joints, TMJ arthroscopic technique, and anatomy and pathology. The rationale and procedures for diagnostic and surgical arthroscopy of the TMJ were presented. Clinical results, indications, contraindications, and complications were outlined. Cooperative research projects were discussed.

It seemed that everyone attending this conference (and those attending two similar conferences in Long Beach, California and in New York) sensed that we were witnesses to the beginning of a major breakthrough in the management of patients with intracapsular temporomandibular joint disorders.

The excitement, enthusiasm, discovery, and controversy that were generated during that time were the stimuli for this book. The authors have included much of the original material presented at the UCLA Symposium as part of this manuscript.

We recognize that all possible TMJ arthroscopic concepts and techniques are not presented here. Many problems are yet to be solved in TMJ arthroscopy. It is hoped that this material will be a stimulus and a reference for further clinical and scientific endeavors.

BRUCE SANDERS
KEN-ICHIRO MURAKAMI
GLENN T. CLARK

Acknowledgments

Dr. Sanders is very grateful for the support, guidance, and co-operative efforts of Drs. Robert Adair, Ron Roth, and Chip Miller of the ENT Section; Drs. Kevin Ehrhart, Todd Grant, Robert Watanabe, and Wayne Christie of the Orthopedic Section; and the Anesthesia Section and operating room nursing staff at Saint John's Hospital and Health Center, Santa Monica, California.

Contents

Introduction / M. Franklin Dolwick ——————— 1

1 Orthopedic Arthroscopy / Kevin M. Ehrhart —— 5

2 Arthroscopic Anatomy / Ken-Ichiro Murakami — 13

3 Operating Room Environment /
Bruce Sanders and Ralph D. Buoncristiani ———— 37

4 Arthroscopic Technique / Bruce Sanders and
Ralph D. Buoncristiani *(Part One)* Ken-Ichiro
Murakami *(Part Two)* ————————————— 47

5 Diagnostic Arthroscopy / Ken-Ichiro
Murakami ——————————————————— 73

6 Surgical Arthroscopy / Bruce Sanders and
Ralph D. Buoncristiani ——————————————— 95

7 Analysis of Arthroscopically Treated TMJ
Derangement and Locking / Glenn T. Clark,
David G. Moody, and Bruce Sanders —————— 115

8 Treatment Planning / John B. Ross,
Bruce Sanders, and Ken-Ichiro Murakami ———— 137

9 Comparative Imaging Study / Carol A. Bibb,
Andrew G. Pullinger, Fernando Baldioceda,
Ken-Ichiro Murakami, and John B. Ross ————— 143

10 Natural History and Pathologic
Progression of Internal Derangements
with Persistent Closed Lock /
Andrew G. Pullinger ——————————————— 159

Introduction /
M. Franklin Dolwick

Arthoscopy is not a new procedure. Professor Kenji Takagi of Tokyo first applied the endoscopic principles of cystoscopy to the examination of the knee joint in 1918. The first writings in the American literature appeared in 1925 when Kreusder reported on the use of the arthroscope in diagnosing meniscal disorders of the knee. It was the Japanese orthopedic community, under the leadership of Takagi, Watanabe, Takeda, and Ikeuchi, however, that developed techniques for performing arthroscopic surgery of the knee.

Enormous technological advances in arthroscopy occurred during the 1970s, and today the use of the arthroscope has dramatically changed the practice of orthopedic surgery. A 1983 membership questionnaire of the American Academy of Orthopedic Surgeons showed that 98 percent used arthroscopy. It is well recognized that arthroscopy has its greatest application in surgery of the knee. The development of small-diameter arthroscopes, however, has expanded its applications to small joints. Clearly, it now seems appropriate to use arthroscopic procedures on the temporomandibular joint (TMJ).

Preliminary reports of outstanding, in fact almost unbelievable, results have stimulated a rush of interest and activity in TMJ arthroscopic surgery. Suddenly the trend is to criticize open TMJ surgery, especially when compared to arthroscopic surgery. But neither criticism of open TMJ surgery nor the enthusiasm for arthroscopy has been based on solid scientific data. As a result of these experiences, many questions arise that will be addressed in this chapter; some of these questions will be answered in this book, while others remain unanswerable at this time.

The first and possibly most important question is whether TMJ arthroscopic surgery should be considered a research procedure. The answer is both yes and no. On the one hand, if rigid scientific principles of research (i.e., systematic study and investigation to discover or establish facts) are applied, then arthroscopy of the TMJ should be considered research. On the other hand, several extensive clinical experiences have been reported that clearly show beneficial results with TMJ arthroscopy. These clinical reports combined with the extensive excellent experiences in using arthroscopy on other joints have led to an acceptance of TMJ arthroscopy by clinicians, and it therefore should not be considered research. Many questions remain unanswered, however, and more research is needed to clarify the role of TMJ arthroscopy in the management of TMJ patients.

The results observed with TMJ arthroscopy challenge our existing concepts of the pathology associated with internal derangement. If simple lavage and lysis of adhesions within the upper joint space significantly decrease pain and improve joint mobility, then disk position and form may not be as important as we previously thought. If disk position and form are not important, then how do we explain the observed pain and dysfunction? The pathologies currently in vogue are synovitis and/or adhesions. Are these observations real or simply a convenient explanation?

The results that have been observed with TMJ arthroscopy have been excellent, but the follow-up periods are short, and little is known yet about long-term results. Certainly, the experiences of orthopedic surgery in other joints indicate that many patients receive good long-term results with simple procedures.

The indications for TMJ arthroscopy are not precise. Some clinicians suggest that all TMJ patients, regardless of their pathology, are candidates and will benefit from the procedure, while other clinicians believe that specific groups of patients (e.g., those with painful limitations of motion) benefit the most. As the results of procedures are examined more closely, the indications for TMJ arthroscopy will become more precise and the outcomes more predictable.

Another important question is, When is it appropriate to intervene arthroscopically? Traditionally, surgical intervention is reserved until late in the course of the problem and not until other therapies have failed. The experiences with arthroscopy in orthopedic surgery have led orthopedic surgeons to use surgical intervention earlier, which is likely to prove true for TMJ arthroscopy as well. When to intervene must be determined, however, through careful investigation.

Although the benefits of therapeutic arthroscopy seem apparent, questions remain about the indications for diagnostic arthroscopy. Observations of arthroscopy within the joint are exciting, interesting, and certainly different from traditional observations, but their significance is not fully known. Diagnostic arthroscopy is an adjunct to (not a substitute for) a complete history and physical examination and appropriate radiographic studies (e.g., tomograms, arthrograms, magnetic resonance imaging [MRI]).

Arthroscopic TMJ surgery is not without potential complications. It is technically difficult, but not impossible. The surgeon should not enter into this adventure halfway. Knowledge of the temporomandibular joint is essential, and basic arthroscopic skills must be mastered before progressing to even the simplest surgical manipulation.

Finally, arthroscopic surgery should not replace sound clinical judgment. It will not solve all TMJ problems and should not be perceived as a panacea. In spite of these concerns, I believe that TMJ arthroscopy will revolutionize the approach to TMJ therapy. Its future is limited only by our imaginations.

1 Orthopedic Arthroscopy / Kevin M. Ehrhart

History of Arthroscopy

Over the last ten years, arthroscopy has become the most important advance in orthopedic surgery. Today, at orthopedic meetings throughout the country, it is the most widely discussed area in orthopedics, and there are monthly meetings throughout the country that deal with very specific applications of the procedure. It appears that throughout orthopedic surgery the topic of discussion is arthroscopy.

The founder of arthroscopy was Dr. Kenji Takagi of the University of Tokyo. In 1918, Dr. Takagi performed the first arthroscopy, on the knee of a corpse. In 1937, Dr. Takagi presented his work to an international orthopedic symposium in Paris. His work was poorly accepted and thought to have no clinical relevance. Over the next 20 years, there were no significant advances in arthroscopy.

In 1957, Dr. Masaki Watanabe, the protege of Dr. Takagi, introduced a prototype arthroscope. Simultaneously, he published his *Atlas of Arthroscopy*. The atlas probably had the greatest impact on the advancement of the procedure at that time. From that time on, arthroscopy became more and more accepted. It was certainly not widespread, but it was being used by research workers throughout the world, most notably in Japan and the United States.

The greatest technical problem at this time was the light source. An incandescent lamp placed at the end of the scope was the only way to introduce light directly into the joint, and this was very cumbersome. A very small amount of light could actually be used, and the light bulb on the end of the scope affected viewing.

In the late 1960s and early 1970s, fiberoptic lens sources became available. Up until that point, the use of fiber glass to carry light was known, but the expense was extraordinarily high and therefore prohibitive. In the 1970s, the fiberoptic light source became commercially available. This allowed a marked improvement in the amount of illumination and in the means by which light could be delivered through the flexible fiberoptic cord.

At this time, Dr. Richard O'Connor, who today is considered the "father" of modern arthroscopy, started his arthroscopic practice in the West Covina area of Los Angeles. Dr. O'Connor first became interested in arthroscopy in the late 1960s. In 1971, he went to the University of Tokyo, where he studied with Dr. Watanabe. On his return to California, Dr. O'Connor began doing operative arthroscopy. Until that time, arthroscopy had been used only as a diagnostic tool, never as a therapeutic modality.

Initially, Dr. O'Connor's procedures were quite simple, consisting of the removal of loose bodies and synovial biopsies. In 1974, however, he introduced the operative arthroscope. This arthroscope allowed an operative instrument to be introduced directly through the cannula that contained the arthroscope so that certain surgical procedures, such as meniscectomies, could be carried out. Though no longer used today, the operative arthroscope ushered in the beginning of the age of operative arthroscopy in the United States.

During the rest of the 1970s, arthroscopy continued to be actively, though not widely, accepted. The major obstacle to its acceptance was the academic community. Teaching centers were very slow to accept arthroscopy—in fact, they were initially so set against the idea that they considered it quackery. This obstinacy was based on several significant and accurate attitudes: one, arthroscopy was new, and nothing new was initially accepted widely at the university level; two, arthroscopy originated outside the university setting, which made the academic world somewhat reluctant to accept it; three, arthroscopy did not have adequate means of internal control by which to evaluate itself. The patient's diagnosis was made by the operating surgeon, the procedure was carried out by the operating surgeon, and no one else could see or judge the results. Four, it was difficult to learn and teach arthroscopy, since arthroscopy was a "one-man job."

In the early 1980s, these attitudes changed dramatically. Many believe the most important reason for the change was the introduction and widespread use of the TV camera and monitor. This, more than anything else, changed arthroscopy from a "cult" to a standard of therapy in orthopedic communities. The TV allowed tremendous advances. First, there was much better visualization. The details of the pathology present were much clearer and much more readily seen. In the hands of an expert arthroscopist, direct visualization was quite clear, but to the "average" arthroscopist, the TV presented a dramatic improvement. Second, other members of the operating team could now "participate" in the procedure and become involved. Before, they could not see what was going on—the room was darkened—which resulted in a lackadaisical atmosphere that affected everyone. Third, the camera allowed the surgeon to be more comfortable while performing the procedure and therefore made it much easier to use instruments to perform "therapeutic arthroscopy" (i.e., operative arthroscopy). Fourth, with TV documentation, the findings were now readily available. Not only could still photographs be produced, but TV viewing was possible. Fifth, the TV camera made it much easier to teach arthroscopy to new orthopedists.

Today, arthroscopy is no longer a cult—it is the basic means of operative therapy for most surgical pathology in the knee, and it is becoming a major means of therapeutic intervention for the shoulder, the elbow, and the ankle. Arthroscopy has been carried out in the wrist in the metacarpophalangeal joints, and now, as oral and maxillofacial surgeons such as Drs. Sanders and Murakami have shown, it is a viable treatment, both for diagnostic and therapeutic purposes, for the temporomandibular joint.

Less than ten years ago, arthroscopy was done by only a few well-trained orthopedists. Today, it is done by almost every orthopedist, and it is a standard part of training programs for every orthopedic resident. Arthroscopy has not only become accepted, it has become the standard of treatment in most communities.

What Is Arthroscopy?

Arthroscopy is a composite of two Greek words: *arthros,* meaning "a joint," and *scopien,* meaning "to view." In essence, arthroscopy is simply a means of looking directly into a joint. Arthroscopy is therefore the visualization of a potentially expandable, well-confined joint. It can be any joint—the knee, the shoulder, or the temporomandibular joint. Arthroscopy has two main indications: first, to help in diagnosing a problem that cannot accurately be determined without direct visualization—diagnostic arthroscopy; second, to render a means of therapeutic intervention—operative arthroscopy.

The diagnostic and therapeutic indications for each specific joint are learned with time. Arthroscopy uses the same basic principles and basic instruments, regardless of which joint is involved. The same principles apply to large joints, such as the knee and shoulder, as to smaller joints, such as the wrist and temporomandibular joint (TMJ).

Instrumentation

The *arthroscope* is actually quite a simple instrument. It is essentially nothing more than a long tube with a magnification lens at one end, through which a light source and an irrigating solution are passed. The ocular piece allows either for direct visualization via the surgeon's eye or for a coupling of the arthroscope to a TV camera. Next to the ocular end of the arthroscope is the attachment for the fiberoptic light source. The far end of the arthroscope is the terminal end of the fiberoptic bundles through which illumination is directly delivered. This arrangement allows very high-intensity illumination to be delivered.

The terminal end of the arthroscope can have a variety of lenses, which can be angled at various degrees to help in visualization. The standard arthroscope used today in orthopedics has a 30° angulation. This provides a much increased area of visualization than a direct 0° scope.

The arthroscope is housed within the *cannula,* which is nothing more than a sheath by which the arthroscope is delivered into the joint and by which the irrigating fluid is introduced into the joint. In orthopedics, all cannulas are the same length. The width varies in orthopedics from 2.7 mm to 5.0 mm. Which cannula and arthroscope to use depends entirely on the surgeon's demands and the size of the joint. A larger cannula and scope allow for greater visualization and more ease in the delivery of irrigating solution. The decision is limited, however, by the size of the joint in question.

The *trochar* is used to introduce the cannula or sheath directly into the joint. It may have either a sharp or a dull end.

The *irrigation system* is an extremely important component of arthroscopy. It has three main functions: first, it allows the joint to be insufflated, that is, expanded beyond its normal size for better visualization and ease of instrumentation in performing therapeutic arthroscopy. Second, the continuous flow of irrigation (usually normal saline or lactated Ringer's) allows removal of joint debris (blood, etc.), which may obscure visualization. The majority of problems encountered during arthroscopy have to do with poor visualization secondary to retained debris within the joint. Third, the irrigation solution reduces the risk of infection. Arthroscopy, whether it be of the shoulder, the knee, or the TMJ, is not always a strictly sterile procedure in the truest sense of the word. The many instruments, changing of the cameras, changing of the arthroscopes, and so on can result in occasional unnoted breaks in sterility. The constant high flow of irrigation to the joint therefore diminishes the risk of infection. The irrigation system therefore helps to fulfill the surgical axiom "the solution to pollution is dilution."

The *solution* used in irrigating the joint is most commonly normal saline, although recent studies have suggested that lactated Ringer's is much more appropriate physiologically and may result in less reactive synovitis to the joint itself. Obviously, the amount of solution used depends on the size of the joint and on the length of the procedure. In temporomandibular joint arthroscopy, the total amount of solution used is dramatically less than the amount used in knee arthroscopy. The irrigation solution may be delivered either by hydrostatic forces (sterile bags of solution hung from high sources that drain into the joint) or by direct, careful infusion into the joint.

In many arthroscopies, there is need for an *efflux system.* The efflux system is nothing more than a large needle or cannula through which the fluid drains by gravity out of the insufflated joint.

Many instruments are used in operative arthroscopy. Although arthroscopy may involve joints of different sizes, from as small as the metacarpophalangeal joint of the finger or the temporomandibular joint to as large as the shoulder, the instruments are all basically the same. The scale and size, however, may be quite different.

The *hook* (or *probe*) is the most important instrument used. It is the basic instrument for performing a diagnostic arthroscopy and often has major importance in therapeutic arthroscopy. The "hook" extends one's "feel" within the joint. It allows the arthroscopist to look beyond what might be seen directly and to "palpate" various structures. The manual dexterity needed to use the probe is the basis for all the manual dexterity in arthroscopic surgery. Certainly, the probe is the instrument that needs to be mastered initially.

Basket forceps, in various sizes, shapes, and angles, are the instruments used to "do the work." It takes time and patience to learn how to use these instruments intra-articularly. The basic method employed in the use of all of these instruments, especially the baskets, is *triangulation.* Triangulation is the process by which the arthroscopist proprioceptively brings together two instruments from different angles to a third point by looking at a fourth period, the TV. One of the most important assets in mastering this procedure is patience. Triangulation is a difficult and frustrating procedure to learn, but with time it can be mastered.

The *mechanized shaver* is used quite extensively in orthopedic surgery. It allows loose tissue to be debrided, solution to be aspirated, and the joint to be vacuumed. There are many different "heads," which in different sizes can be applied to the shaver to perform the necessary function. The device consists of a revolving blade within a cannula. The tissue is sucked into the mouth of the cannula through suction applied to the shaver itself. The revolving blade, or teeth, amputates the tissue and aspirates it away. It is a very helpful and important instrument for all arthroscopic surgeries.

The last major component necessary for successful arthroscopy is the *nursing team.* It cannot be stressed enough how important the nursing team is for the success of arthroscopic surgery. Arthroscopy cannot be done without a team that is totally in tune with the procedure. Arthroscopy is difficult. It requires nurses to relearn an entire set of instruments. It requires quite a bit of activity during the procedure, including setting up, suctioning, constantly changing irrigating solutions, moving the camera, adjusting the light source, and so on. If the nurses do not feel they are part of the team, they will become frustrated and lose interest, and the arthroscopist will find it impossible to perform the procedure. It is therefore important for every surgeon who performs arthroscopic surgery to have a team with whom he or she works routinely.

Applications of Arthroscopy

In orthopedic surgery, the wealth of experience has centered on knee surgery. Knee arthroscopy accounts for greater than 95 percent of all orthopedic arthroscopies. The knee shares many anatomical similarities with the temporomandibular joint. It is therefore natural to try to apply some of the clinical experience gained in knee arthroscopy to TMJ arthroscopy.

A quick review of the basic anatomy of the knee reveals many similarities between it and the temporomandibular joint. The knee consists of "two joints," the bicompartmental femorotibial joint and the patellofemoral joint. The patellofemoral joint, which in orthopedics is a major source of problems, does not have an analog in the temporomandibular joint. The femorotibial joint is very analogous, however.

The *femoral condyles* are covered with hyaline cartilage. The femoral condyle in turn articulates with the tibial plateau, which is also covered with articular hyaline cartilage. Along the periphery of both the medial and lateral compartments is the fibrocartilaginous *meniscus*. The meniscus functions, first, to distribute weight evenly from the round femoral condyle to the flat-shaped tibial plateau; second, to stabilize the joint; and third, to absorb energy. It is a primary source of arthroscopic pathology within the knee.

The entire joint is surrounded by the *capsule*. There is an expansion of the capsule above the joint known as the suprapatellar *fossa* or *pouch*. The entire joint, except for the cartilage, is lined with synovium.

Problems can arise in any of these multiple areas. The etiology of these problems may be secondary to (1) trauma; (2) congenital anomaly; (3) degeneration; (4) inflammation; or (5) infectious processes. Classification therefore may be based on the etiology or the anatomy itself. Presented below is an anatomical classification of arthroscopic pathology and how this pathology may be amenable to arthroscopic surgery.

Synovial Lesions

Synovitis, whether it is primary, as seen in rheumatoid arthritis, or secondary, as seen with trauma, infection, or degeneration, is a very significant problem. It leads to pain, swelling, and loss of motion. Treatment is two-pronged. First, treat the causative agent; second, treat the synovitis itself. Often this can be done through a conservative approach with medications and therapy, but sometimes it requires surgical intervention. In the past, this has necessitated a synovectomy via an arthrotomy. This was a major procedure in which there was a significant morbidity. Today, this procedure is done relatively atraumatically via arthroscopy as an outpatient procedure, and there is a dramatic difference in the postoperative course.

The mechanized shaver is the instrument by which the synovium is resected. Removing the synovium in this case greatly enhances joint function and eases the patient's pain. At the same time, there is no arthrotomy, and mobilization may be begun almost immediately. This eliminates one of the major sources of morbidity from arthrotomy—adhesions and loss of motion.

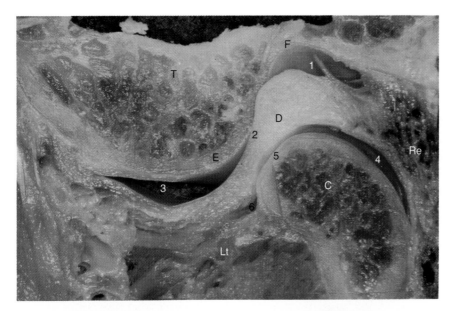

FIGURE 2-1 / Sagittal section of left TMJ. The upper joint cavity consists of the posterior synovial pouch (1), the intermediate space (2), and the anterior synovial recess (3). The lower joint cavity consists of the posterior synovial pouch (4), the intermediate space (5), and the anterior synovial pouch (6). T, temporal bone; F, mandibular fossa; E, articular eminence; D, articular disk; C, condylar head; Re, retrodiscal pad; Lt, lateral pterygoid muscle. (From Murakami K, Hoshino K: Regional anatomical nomenclature and arthroscopic terminology in human temporomandibular joint. Okajimas Folia Anat Jpn 58:745-760, 1982.)

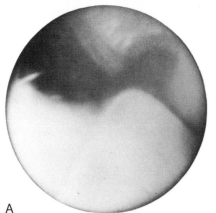

A

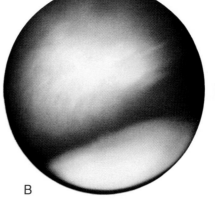

B

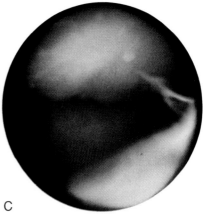

C

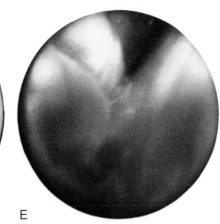

D

E

FIGURE 2-2 / Arthroscopic construction of upper and lower joint cavities. Each arthroscopic photograph indicates anatomical landmarks in each subsided compartment, *A*, upper posterior synovial pouch; *B*, intermediate space; *C*, anterior synovial recess; *D*, lower posterior synovial pouch; *E*, anterior synovial pouch.

Arthroscopic Subdivision: Anatomy and Pathology

The arthroscopic views of each subdivided compartment in the upper and lower joint cavities reveal individual anatomical features. Some pathological abnormalities are characteristic of a particular anatomical location. Hyperemia and congestion on the synovial membrane, or synovitis, is seen at the posterior synovial pouch in the upper joint cavity, whereas fibrous adhesion is noted frequently at the anterior synovial recess. Extensive or localized fibrillation and chondromalacia may occur on the articular eminence at the intermediate space.

Each of the following sections shows upper and lower compartment subdivisions with arthroscopic, gross, and microscopic anatomical views. Representative pathological abnormalities are also illustrated for each compartment. The arthroscopic approach to these anatomical views is described in the section on technique (Chap. 4). For ease in explanation, anatomical features are described in the order of our preferred method of examination: upper posterior synovial pouch, upper anterior synovial recess, and intermediate space in the upper joint cavity, followed by investigation of the lower posterior and anterior synovial pouches (see the sequence of views in the schematic drawings). For convenience, description of the intermediate space in the lower joint cavity is included in the illustrations of the anterior and posterior synovial pouch.

Upper Posterior Synovial Pouch (Fig. 2-3)

The synovial membrane is an arthroscopic anatomical landmark, which appears soft, occurs posteriorly, and reflects upward to the mandibular fossa (Fig. 2–4). From the lateral aspect, a number of synovial folds are observed on the surface of the synovial membrane; they disappear when the disk slides anteriorly (Fig. 2–5). Although it is difficult to find a clear transitional line from the articular surface in front of the synovial membrane, both structures are easily distinguished. Many translucent vascular patterns are seen on the surface of the synovial membrane (Fig. 2–6 and 2–7).

The surface view of the synovial membrane changes in response to disk malposition. For instance, patients with irreducible anterior disk displacement usually demonstrate stretching of the synovial membrane that changes little with jaw movement (Fig. 2–8).

Rupture involving tearing of the posterior disk attachment is usually associated with moderate to severe synovitis. Localized redness and congestion are occasionally observed on the posterior aspects of the mandibular fossa in association with this disorder.

Histologically, mild synovitis with granulative changes affects the synovial membrane.

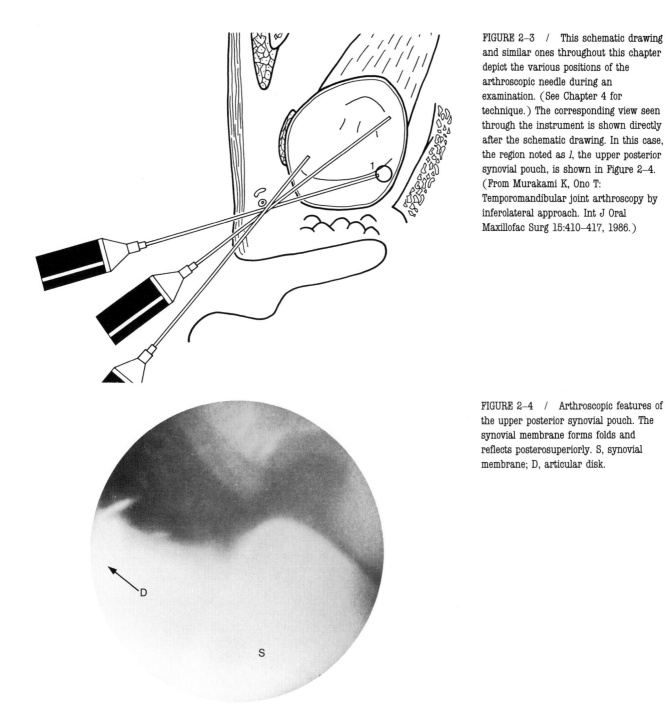

FIGURE 2–3 / This schematic drawing and similar ones throughout this chapter depict the various positions of the arthroscopic needle during an examination. (See Chapter 4 for technique.) The corresponding view seen through the instrument is shown directly after the schematic drawing. In this case, the region noted as *1*, the upper posterior synovial pouch, is shown in Figure 2–4. (From Murakami K, Ono T: Temporomandibular joint arthroscopy by inferolateral approach. Int J Oral Maxillofac Surg 15:410–417, 1986.)

FIGURE 2–4 / Arthroscopic features of the upper posterior synovial pouch. The synovial membrane forms folds and reflects posterosuperiorly. S, synovial membrane; D, articular disk.

FIGURE 2–5 / Another arthroscopic view of the upper posterior synovial pouch. The synovial membrane is stretched anteriorly (left) by a positional change in the disk caused by opening of the jaw. At the posterior end of the synovial membrane, the underlying posterior diskal attachment can be seen. S, synovial membrane; Ca, medial capsular wall inner lined by the synovial membrane; Po, posterior diskal attachment to the mandibular fossa (F).

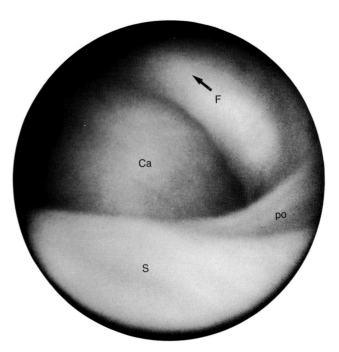

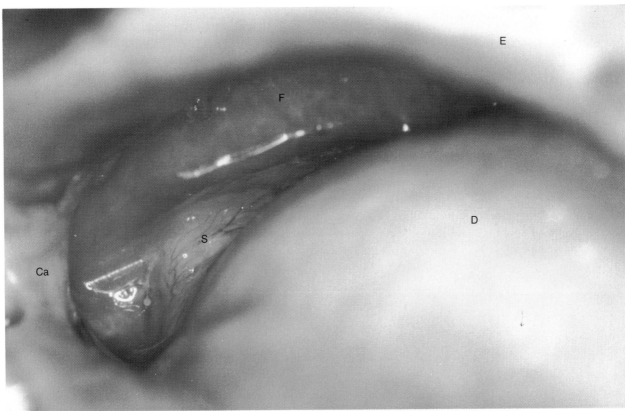

FIGURE 2–6 / The upper posterior synovial pouch, viewed from an anteromedial direction. E, articular eminence; D, articular disk; F, mandibular fossa; S, synovial membrane (distributed in the pouch); Ca, medial capsule. (From Murakami K, Hoshino K: Regional anatomical nomenclature and arthroscopic terminology in human temporomandibular joint. Okajimas Folia Anat Jpn 58:745–760, 1982.)

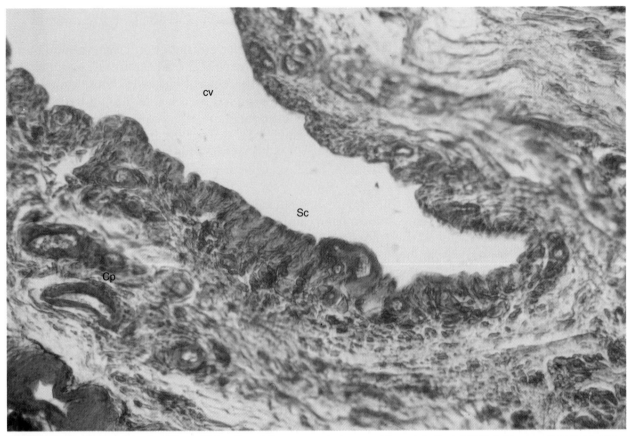

FIGURE 2-7 / Photomicrograph of the sagittal section of the upper posterior synovial pouch in the left TMJ. A few rows of synovial cells line the surface of the synovial membrane. Many capillaries are found among the superficial synovial cell layer and in the subsynovial connective tissue. Cv, upper joint cavity; Sc, synovial cell layer; Cp, capillaries. (Courtesy of Murakami K, Hoshino K: Department of Anatomy at Kyoto University Faculty of Medicine.)

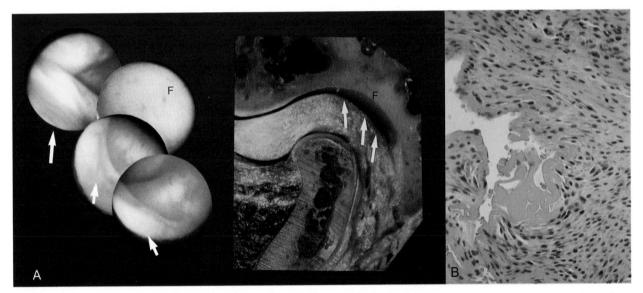

FIGURE 2-8 / A, Arthroscopic composite photograph from a patient with anterior disk displacement with closed lock. Arrows indicate the stretched posterior attachment covered by the synovial membrane, which shows signs of inflammation. The inset indicates the location of arthroscopic view in a cadaver specimen. F, mandibular fossa. B, Histopathological section taken from the same example. The findings show mild inflammatory cell infiltration.

Upper Anterior Synovial Recess (Fig. 2–9)

The lower surface of the articular eminence and the synovial membrane lining in the anterior aspect of the recess are the usual visible anatomical landmarks in this region (Fig. 2–10). Less translucent vascularity is seen on the synovial membrane than in the posterior pouch. The articular eminence and the synovial membrane adjacent to the anterior aspect of the articular disk closely oppose each other (Figs. 2–11 and 2–12). When the jaw opens, this recess increases in size because of the anterior translation of the disk (Fig. 2–13).

In anterior disk displacement, this recess also increases with some deformation, and the anteromedial groove may be observed in the transitional area between the disk and the synovial membrane, just below the articular eminence.

Hyperemia, congestion, microscopic areas of bleeding on the synovial membrane, and mild to moderate synovitis are observed in patients with internal derangement with closed jaw locking. These pathological changes occasionally are accompanied by fibrillation on the articular eminence (Fig. 2–14A).

Fibrous adhesion is sometimes detected in this recess in patients with persistent closed locking. The state and extent of the pathological condition range from mild to severe (Fig. 2–14B).

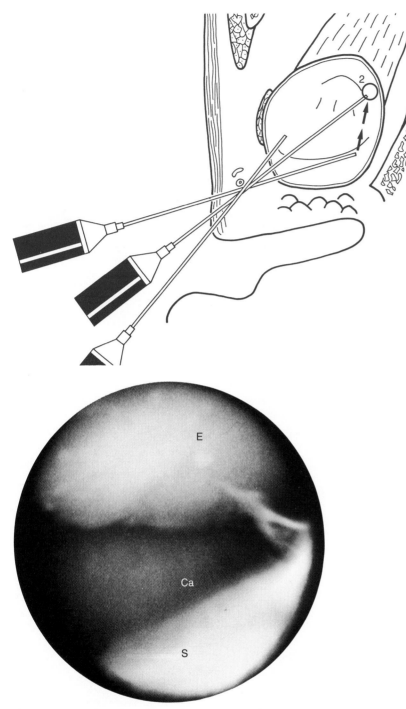

FIGURE 2–9 / Schematic drawing depicting view of the upper anterior synovial recess (2).

FIGURE 2–10 / The anterior synovial recess, as seen from a posterolateral direction. E, articular eminence; Ca, anteromedial capsular wall, lined with the synovial membrane (S).

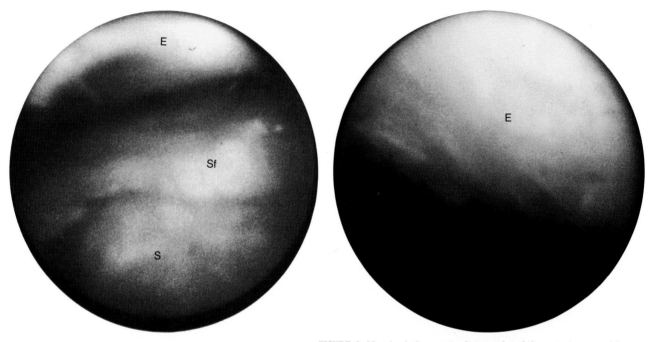

FIGURE 2–11 / Arthroscopic photographs of the anterior synovial recess. E, articular eminence; S, synovial membrane; Sf, synovial flange.

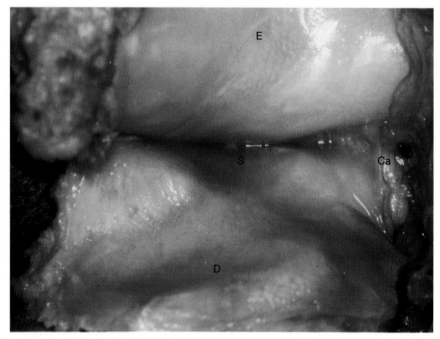

FIGURE 2–12 / The upper joint cavity of the left TMJ, opened from the back (lateral aspect is on left of picture). The anterior synovial recess is viewed in the anterior aspect. E, articular eminence; S, synovial membrane; Ca, medial capsule; D, articular disk. (Courtesy of Murakami K, Hoshino K: Department of Anatomy at Kyoto University Faculty of Medicine.)

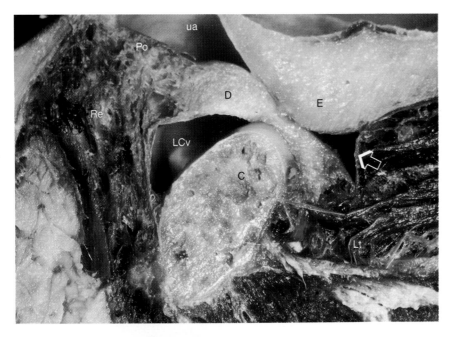

FIGURE 2–13 / Sagittal section of the right TMJ with the jaw open. The size of the upper anterior synovial recess is increased (*arrow*). UCv, upper joint cavity; LCv, lower joint cavity; E, articular eminence; Lt, lateral pterygoid muscle; D, articular disk; C, condylar head; Re, retrodiscal pad; Po, posterior discal attachment. (Courtesy of Murakami K, Bibb C, Baldioceda F: Temporomandibular Joint Laboratory, UCLA Dental Research Institute.)

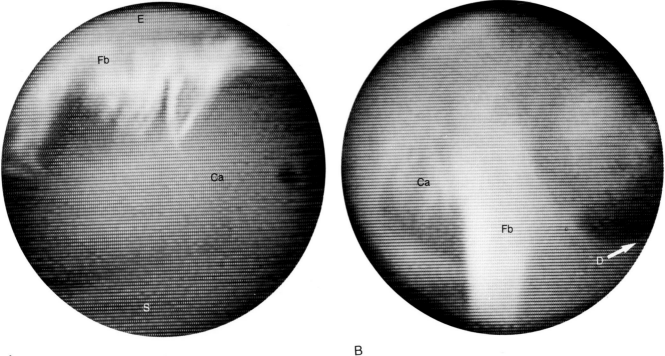

A

B

FIGURE 2–14 / *A*, Chondromalacia in the right TMJ. Inflammatory changes involve the upper anterior synovial recess. The synovial membrane and wall are reddened and show hyperemic changes. E, articular eminence; Fb, fibrillation; Ca, capsular wall; S, synovial membrane. *B*, Fibrous adhesion in the left TMJ. Severe fibrous adhesion is detected in the anterior recess. Fb, Fibrous adhesion; Ca, capsular wall. Arrow indicates orientation to the disk.

Intermediate Space in the Upper Joint Cavity (Fig. 2–15)

This intermediate space is located in the central articulating zone in the upper joint cavity. The articular surface of the posterior slope of the articular eminence and the upper surface of the articular disk are easy to define (Fig. 2–16). Their surface views look smooth and shiny and appear avascular. Both structures are close together, and the surface of the articular disk looks more whitish. The articular disk slides forward during jaw opening, but the surface view does not alter (Figs. 2–17 and 2–18). Articular surfaces covering the bone and on the articular disk are composed mainly of avascular, fibrous, dense connective tissue with the histological characteristics of fibrocartilage (Fig. 2–19).

The most common pathological change is extensive or localized fibrillation, which is sometimes found on the posterior slope of the articular eminence (Fig. 2–20A). Localized severe fibrillation resembles that of chondromalacia (Fig. 2–20B). Occasionally, extensive fibrillation on the articular disk surface is observed; this indicates surface adhesion. In some cases, severe fibrous adhesion is detected. On the articular eminence, surface roughening and irregularity of the articular cartilage are found.

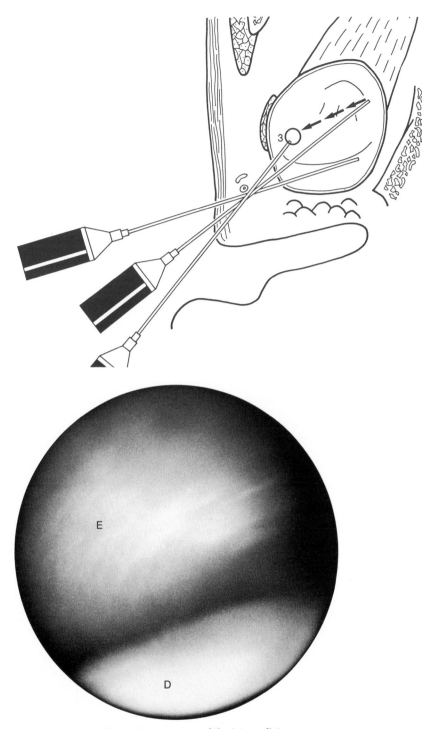

FIGURE 2–15 / Schematic drawing of arthroscopic examination of the intermediate space in the upper joint cavity (3).

FIGURE 2–16 / Arthroscopic appearance of the intermediate space. It consists of articular surfaces on both the temporal component and the articular disk. E, posterior slope of the articular eminence; D, upper surface of the articular disk.

FIGURE 2–17 / The upper joint cavity of the right TMJ has been opened anteriorly. Smooth and shiny articular surfaces of the articular eminence and articular disk can be seen. E, anterior aspect of the articular eminence; D, upper articular surface of the disk; S, synovial membrane distributed in the posterior synovial pouch (*); Ca, medial capsular wall. (From Murakami K, Hoshino K: Regional anatomical nomenclature and arthroscopic terminology in human temporomandibular joint. Okajimas Folia Anat Jpn 58: 745–760, 1982.)

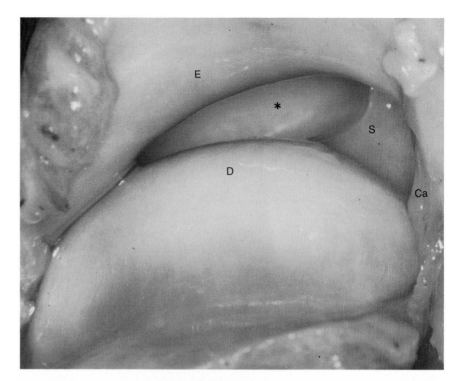

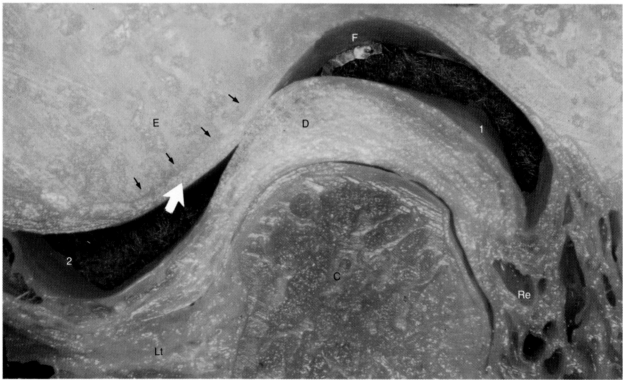

FIGURE 2–18 / Sagittal section of the left TMJ with the jaw slightly open. Large arrow indicates the intermediate space in the upper joint cavity. Small arrows show well-defined soft tissue covering the temporal bone. 1, posterior synovial pouch; 2, anterior recess; E, articular eminence; F, mandibular fossa; D, articular disk; C, condylar head; Re, retrodiskal pad; Lt, lateral pterygoid muscle. (Courtesy of Murakami K, Hoshino K: Department of Anatomy at Kyoto University Faculty of Medicine.)

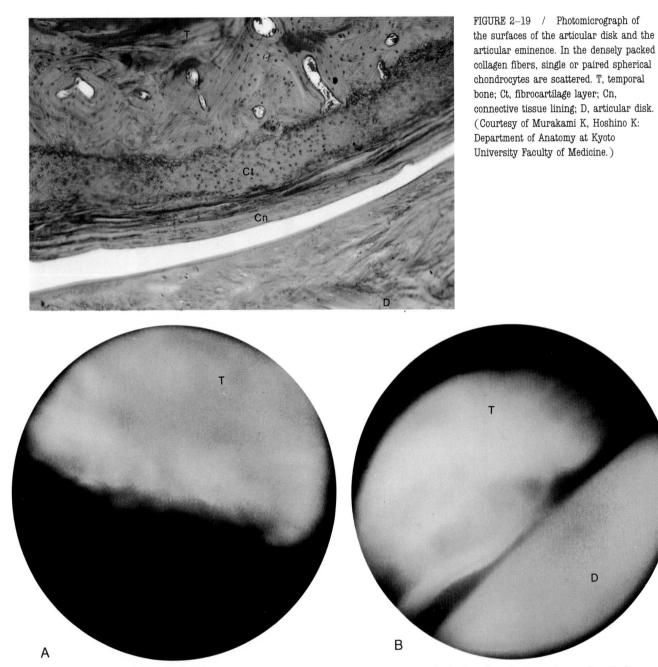

FIGURE 2–19 / Photomicrograph of the surfaces of the articular disk and the articular eminence. In the densely packed collagen fibers, single or paired spherical chondrocytes are scattered. T, temporal bone; Ct, fibrocartilage layer; Cn, connective tissue lining; D, articular disk. (Courtesy of Murakami K, Hoshino K: Department of Anatomy at Kyoto University Faculty of Medicine.)

FIGURE 2–20 / *A*, Extensive fibrillation on the articular eminence. *B*, Chondromalacia is detected on the articular eminence. T, articular eminence; D, articular disk.

Lower Posterior Synovial Pouch (Fig. 2–21)

The posterior surfaces of the mandibular condyle and of the synovial membrane appear opposite each other in this area (Fig. 2–22). The synovial membrane of this portion looks more vascularized because of the blood vessels beneath the retrodiskal pad. The surface view looks softer and similar to the cushionlike appearance; however, a number of synovial foldings appearing in the upper posterior synovial pouch are not detected (Figs. 2–23 and 2–24). The surface view changes little during changes in the position of the disk. The synovial membrane lines the retrodiskal pad, which is composed of loose connective tissues rich in interstitial collagen fibers, a large amount of adipose tissues, abundant arteries, and a venous plexus (Fig. 2–25).

Hyperemia, congestion, and synovitis may be detected on the synovial membrane, and rupture has been observed in cadaver specimens (Fig. 2–26A). The higher portion of the condylar head faces the lower surface of the articular disk (Fig. 2–26B). On the posterior surface of the condyle in this pouch, osteophytes and irregular structures are occasionally found.

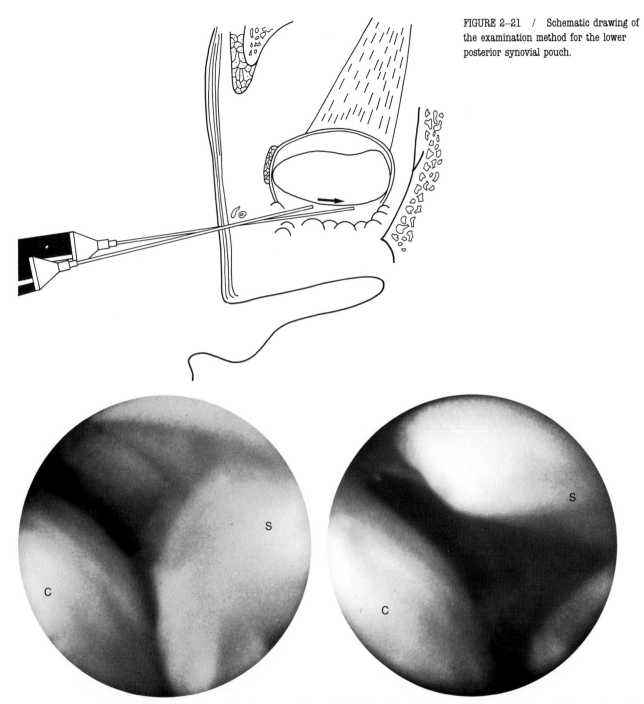

FIGURE 2-21 / Schematic drawing of the examination method for the lower posterior synovial pouch.

FIGURE 2-22 / Lateral arthroscopic views of the lower posterior pouch. *Left*, jaw is opened. *Right*, jaw is closed. The posterior surface of the condylar head and the cushionlike structure of the synovial membrane closely face each other. C, posterior aspect of the condylar head; S, synovial membrane.

FIGURE 2-23 / Surface view of the synovial membrane in the lower posterior pouch. A cushionlike structure is observed. Small capillaries are found throughout the synovial membrane.

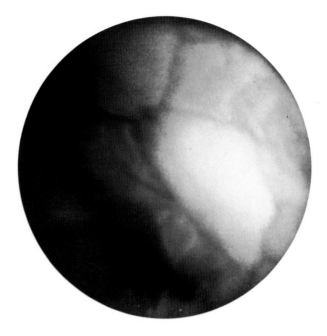

FIGURE 2-24 / Posterior aspect of the lower joint cavity, opened anteriorly. The articular disk (D) is reflected superiorly. Lt, sphenomeniscus portion of the lateral pterygoid muscle, attached to the anterior aspect of the disk; S, synovial membrane distributed in the lower posterior synovial pouch; C, posterior surface of the condylar head. (From Murakami K, Hoshino K: Regional anatomical nomenclature and arthroscopic terminology in human temporomandibular joint. Okajimas Folia Anat Jpn 58:745–760, 1982.)

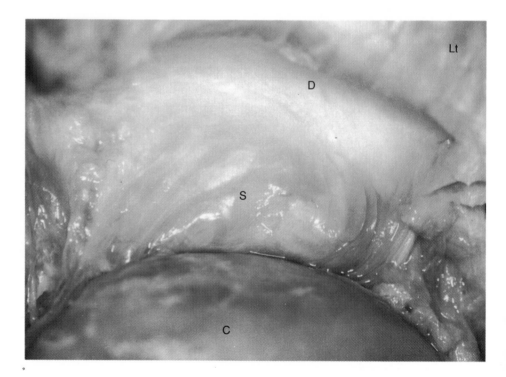

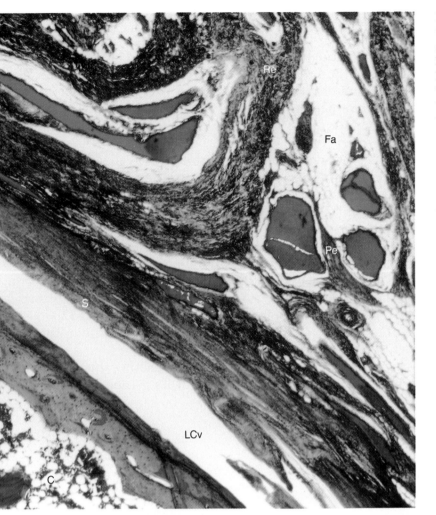

FIGURE 2-25 / Photomicrograph of the sagittal section of the lower posterior synovial pouch of the left TMJ. LCv, lower joint space; Re, retrodiskal pad is lined by the synovial membrane (S), which is facing the posterior surface of the condylar head (C); Fa, adipose tissue; Pl, venous plexus and small arteries. (From Murakami K, Hoshino K: Histological studies on the inner surfaces of the articular cavities of human temporomandibular joints with special reference to arthroscopic observations. Anat Anz 160:167–177, 1985.)

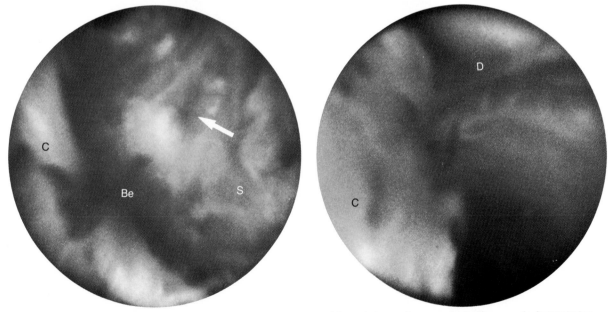

FIGURE 2-26 / Arthroscopic photographs of the lower posterior synovial pouch in a cadaver specimen. The example demonstrates irreducible anterior disk displacement. In the left picture, the arrow indicates the rupturing on the synovial membrane. Synovitis and microbleeding are seen. S, synovial membrane; C, condylar head; Bl, bleeding clot; D, lower surface of the articular disk. (Courtesy of Murakami K, Bibb C, Baldioceda F: Temporomandibular Joint Laboratory, UCLA Dental Research Institute.)

Lower Anterior Synovial Pouch (Fig. 2-27)

This compartment has the least articular space in the TMJ and consists of the anterior aspect of the mandibular condyle head, the synovial membrane, and the anterior part of the lower surface of the articular disk (Fig. 2–28).

The surface of the synovial membrane appears less flexible here than in other regions of the TMJ. Although fine synovial folds are detected, vascularity of the membrane is negligible. Synovial reflection upward toward the lower surface of the articular disk is similar to that in the upper posterior pouch, and the anterior part of the articular disk appears uneven but slightly protuberant. Since no vascularity is seen on the surface of the disk, the transition between these two structures is not easy to identify. The anterior aspect of the condyle appears more smooth and shiny than does the posterior aspect (Fig. 2–29 and 2–30).

When the disk is anteriorly displaced, there is a slight increase in the space in this compartment (Figs. 2–31 and 2–32).

Inflammatory changes of the synovial membrane in this pouch have not been recorded.

Because of clinical difficulties in inspecting this compartment by arthroscopy, little is known about its pathological changes.

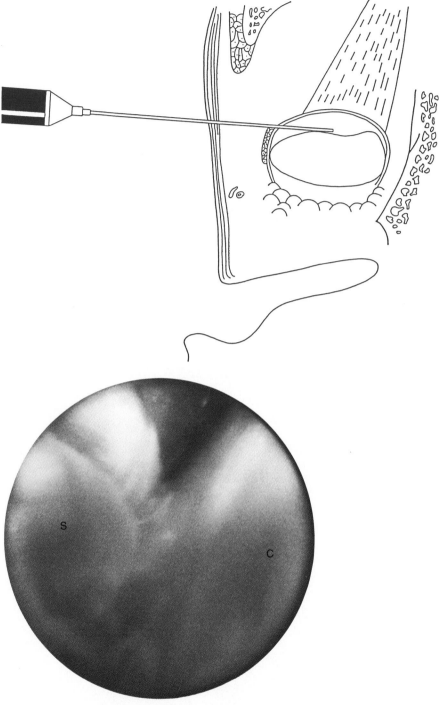

FIGURE 2–27 / Schematic representation of view of the lower anterior synovial pouch.

FIGURE 2–28 / Arthroscopic photograph of the lower anterior synovial pouch. S, synovial membrane; C, condylar head.

FIGURE 2–29 / Macroscopic view of
the anterior aspect of the sagittal section
of the left TMJ. *UCv*, upper joint cavity;
LCv, lower joint cavity. Lower anterior
synovial pouch is indicated by (*). *E*,
articular eminence; *D*, articular disk; *C*,
anterior aspect of the mandibular
condyle; *S*, synovial membrane distributed
in the lower anterior synovial pouch.
(Courtesy of Murakami K, Hoshino K:
Department of Anatomy at Kyoto
University Faculty of Medicine.)

FIGURE 2–30 / Photomicrograph of
the lower anterior synovial pouch (*). *D*,
articular disk; *C*, condylar head of the
mandible; *S*, synovial membrane. Small
capillaries (*Cp*) are seen underneath the
synovial membrane. (Courtesy of
Murakami K, Hoshino K: Department of
Anatomy at Kyoto University Faculty of
Medicine.)

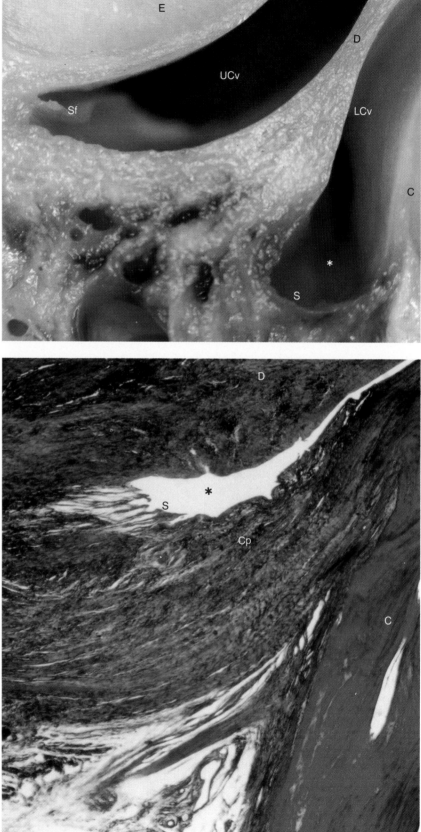

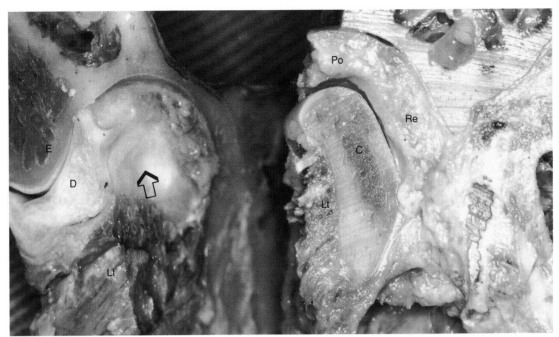

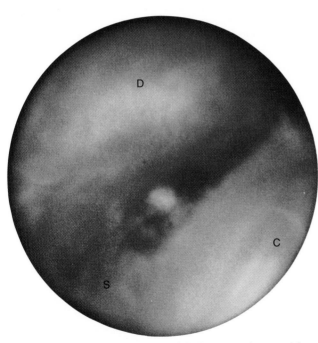

FIGURE 2-31 / Dissected specimen showing irreducible anterior disk displacement. Sagittally sectioned left TMJ was cut in front of the condyle head. The arrow indicates enlargement of the lower anterior synovial pouch due to anterior disk displacement. *E*, articular eminence; *D*, articular disk; *Lt*, lateral pterygoid muscle; *Po*, posterior diskal attachment; *Re*, retrodiskal pad; *C*, condylar head. (Courtesy of Murakami K, Hoshino K: Department of Anatomy at Kyoto University Faculty of Medicine.)

FIGURE 2-32 / Arthroscopic view of the lower anterior synovial pouch in a specimen showing irreducible anterior disk displacement. *D*, lower aspect of the articular disk; *C*, anterior aspect of the mandibular condyle head; *S*, synovial membrane. (Courtesy of Murakami K, Bibb C, Baldioceda F: Temporomandibular Joint Laboratory, UCLA Dental Research Institute.)

Acknowledgment

Much of the anatomical and histological data were collected in the Department of Anatomy at Kyoto University Faculty of Medicine in cooperation with Dr. K. Hoshino.

References

Holmlund A, Hellsing G: Arthroscopy of the temporomandibular joint. An autopsy study. Int J Oral Surg 14:169–175, 1985.

Lutz D, Schwipper V, Fritzemeier CU: Die Endoskopie des Kiefergelenkes—eine neue Untersuchungsmethode. Dtsch Zahnaerztl Z 36:183–186, 1981.

Murakami K, Hoshino K: Regional anatomical nomenclature and arthroscopic terminology in human temporomandibular joints. Okajimas Folia Anat 58:745–760, 1982.

Murakami K, Hoshino K: Histological studies on the inner surfaces of the articular cavities of human temporomandibular joints with special reference to arthroscopic observations. Anat Anz 160:167–177, 1985.

Kino K: Morphological and structural observation of the synovial membranes and their folds relating to the endoscopic findings in the upper cavity of the human temporomandibular joint. J Stomatol Soc Jpn 47:98, 1980 (in Japanese, abstract in English).

Kino K, Ohnishi M, Shioda S, Ichijo T: Morphological observation on the inner surface of the temporomandibular joint: Histological investigation relating to the arthroscopic findings in the upper cavity. Jpn J Oral Surg 27:1379, 1981 (in Japanese).

Murakami K, Ito K: Arthroscopy of the temporomandibular joint: Arthroscopic anatomy and arthroscopic approaches in the human cadaver. Arthroscopy 6:1–13, 1981 (in Japanese, abstract in English).

Ohnishi M: Arthroscopy of the temporomandibular joint. J Stomatol Soc Jpn 42:207–213, 1975 (in Japanese).

3 Operating Room Environment /

Bruce Sanders
Ralph D. Buoncristiani

Surgical Area

TMJ arthroscopy is done on an outpatient basis in the hospital. If diagnostic arthroscopy is followed by arthrotomy, the patient is admitted for postoperative care. Arthroscopy is done in the operating room while the patient is under general anesthesia with nasoendotracheal intubation (Fig. 3–1A-D). The patient is prepared and draped in the same manner as in arthrotomy procedures.

The surgical table should be positioned so that the anesthesiologist is well off to the side of the patient (Fig. 3–1E). The surgeon, assistant surgeon, and scrub nurse should have direct visibility of the monitor (Fig. 3–1F). The arthroscope and camera head should be at the head of the table in a basin within reach of the surgeon (Fig. 3–1G-I). It is essential that the surgeon have a team that he or she repeatedly works with, including an assistant surgeon, arthroscopy scrub nurse, arthroscopy circulating nurse, and anesthesiologist (Fig. 3–1J). It is helpful for the surgeon to do all his/her TMJ arthroscopy procedures in one hospital, preferably one with pre-existing high-quality orthopedic arthroscopy activity. This will ensure expert care of the highly technical arthroscopy equipment and the availability of trained arthroscopy nurses.

TMJ Arthroscopy Instruments and Equipment

Arthroscopy, by its very nature, is a highly equipment-dependent procedure. A basic understanding of how the arthroscope, cameras, and associated equipment work and how this equipment interconnects is vital to ensure smooth diagnostic and surgical arthroscopic procedures and to prevent or correct problems.

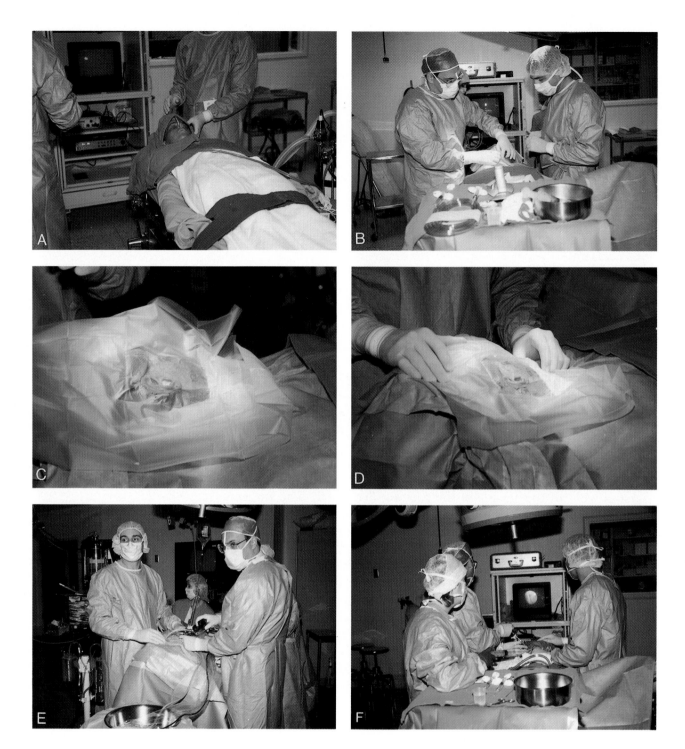

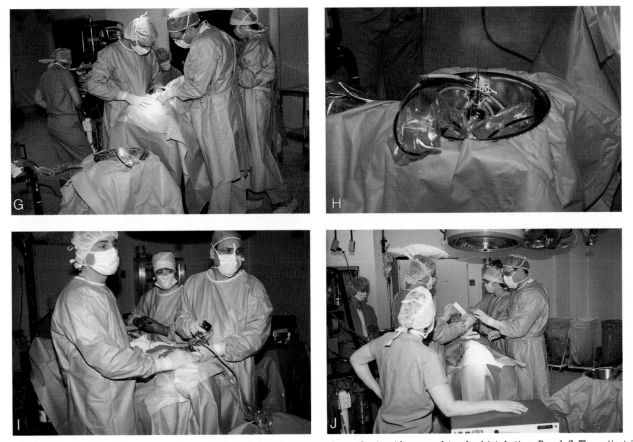

FIGURE 3–1 / Operating room environment. *A*, Patient is given general anesthesia with nasoendotracheal intubation. *B* and *C*, The patient is prepared and draped as for TMJ arthrotomy procedures. *D*, The mouth is covered with a plastic drape, placed so that the assistant surgeon may place a thumb intraorally, without "contaminating," to manipulate the mandible. *E*, The anesthesiologist should be well off to the side of the surgical table so that the surgeon and assistant surgeon may have access to operate and exchange positions during right and left TMJ arthroscopies. *F*, It is essential that the surgeon, assistant surgeon, and scrub nurse have direct visibility of the monitor. *G*, *H*, and *I*, The arthroscope and VCR camera should be at the head of the table in a sterile draped basin within the reach of the surgeon. *J*, Efficient, high-quality TMJ arthroscopy requires a team that works together frequently.

An arthroscope is basically a rigid metal tube with magnifying lenses at both ends. Within the metal cylinder there is a series of lenses that transmit the image from the objective lens (joint end) to the ocular lens (eye or camera end) (Fig. 3–2). Around these lenses are light-conducting glass fibers arranged so that they provide even illumination of the field of view within the joint (Fig. 3–3).

Arthroscopy of the temporomandibular joint requires the use of a small-diameter arthroscope. We have used arthroscopes with diameters ranging from 1.9 mm to 2.7 mm (Fig. 3–4). These arthroscopes allow less traumatic entry to the joint and easier positioning within the joint compartment than arthroscopes with larger diameters. On the other hand, smaller arthroscopes are more easily damaged by inadvertent flexing of the shaft and have a narrower field of view (Fig. 3–5). Wider-angle lenses are beneficial to gain a broad viewing field (Fig. 3–6), but they may create some image distortion and reduce illumination of the apparent field. Lens systems used by arthroscopes employed for small-joint arthroscopy allow anywhere from 55° to 79° of view from the end of the arthroscope. This is variable depending on the optics and the medium through which the arthroscope is viewing (air versus irrigation media within the joint). Angled arthroscopes allow this view to be in a forward oblique direction, which can be helpful in viewing instruments or gaining visualization to lateral recesses of the joint (Fig. 3–7).

Because of the small size of TMJ arthroscopes, an intense light source is necessary to provide adequate illumination. High-intensity sources have provided a cold and powerful beam that can be transmitted with minimal loss through high-quality fiberoptic light cables (Fig. 3–8).

Visualization can be accomplished by looking directly through the eye piece on the arthroscope. With the advent of small video cameras, it has become more convenient and advantageous to use this camera to receive the image for inspection on a video monitor (Fig. 3–9).

There are several advantages to using a video camera. There is less chance of contamination of the surgical field and arthroscope. The image is enlarged on the monitor screen. The surgeon's comfort is enhanced as the operator does not have to stoop or bend to maintain eye position behind the arthroscope. Both the surgeon and the assistant are able to watch the arthroscopic field and to participate in the evaluation of surgical pathology seen in the joint. Documentation of surgical findings and surgical procedures by means of video tape recordings can be made.

In the past, ¾-inch video tape was preferred for tape recording because of its higher-quality image recording. Good-quality ½-inch (Beta or VHS) industrial-grade video tape machines are now available and provide an adequate and less expensive means of documentation.

The functional arthroscope assembly is made up of a sheath/inflow assembly, or cannula, and the arthroscope itself. The sheath is a

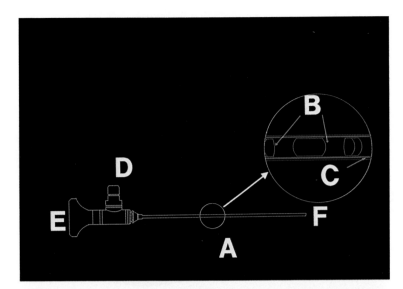

FIGURE 3–2   /   Simplified construction of an arthroscope. *A*, rigid metal tube; *B*, rod lens system for image transmittance; *C*, light-conducting glass fibers; *D*, light source connection; *E*, ocular lens; *F*, objective lens.

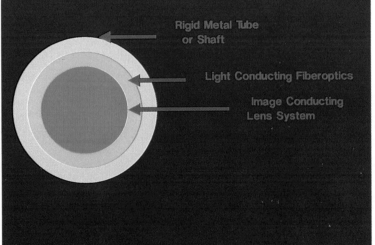

FIGURE 3–3   /   Cross-sectional representation of an arthroscope showing light-conducting glass fibers arranged around the lens system.

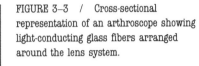

FIGURE 3–4   /   Arthroscopic equipment used for the temporomandibular joint. Top to bottom: blunt obturator, pyramidal obturator, sharp trochar, canula, reinforced canula, 1.9-mm 25-degree arthroscope, 1.9-mm 5-degree arthroscope.

FIGURE 3-5 / An impaired image showing a dark crescent
resulting from bending of the arthroscope.

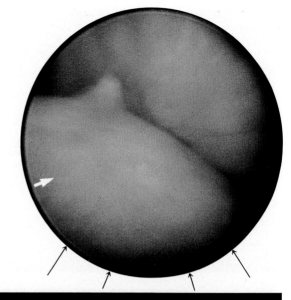

FIGURE 3-6 / The angle of vision of
an arthroscope (wide-angle lens).

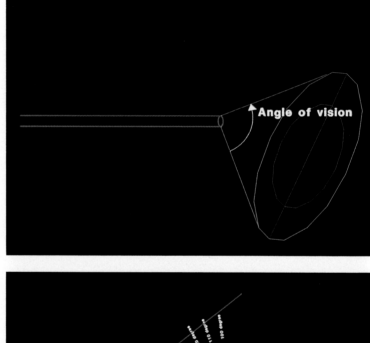

FIGURE 3-7 / Arthroscopes are
available in various angles. Angled
viewing direction is offset from the long
axis of the arthroscope. This allows
viewing in a forward oblique direction
(e.g., 5 degrees or 25 degrees).

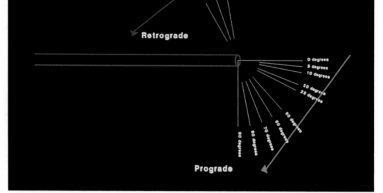

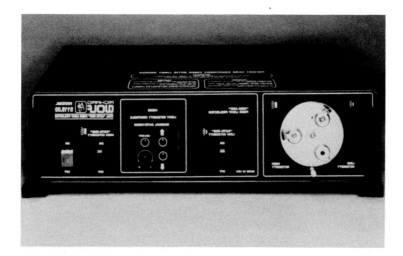

FIGURE 3–8 / Wolf high-intensity Dual Auto-Iris Fiberlight projector light source. Light level is automatically regulated via an intermediate connection between the video camera and the monitor. (Courtesy of Richard Wolf Medical Instrument Corp.)

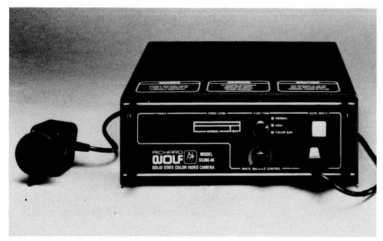

FIGURE 3–9 / Wolf half-inch CCD video camera system. (Courtesy of Richard Wolf Medical Instrument Corp.)

smooth, thin-walled, rigid metal tube that comes in several shapes and diameters. The sheath allows for exchanging of trochars and the introduction of the arthroscope by way of a single puncture. The sheath also provides a locking mechanism to stabilize either the scope or the trochars. The locking mechanism both stabilizes the trochar or scope and provides a seal to prevent backflow of irrigation fluid. A port, or stopcock, allows fluids to be infused into the sheath. Space between the arthroscope and the sheath provides a route for flow of irrigation into the joint (Fig. 3–10).

Trochars and obturators are provided in a variety of designs with both blunt and sharp ends to allow sheath assembly placement and movement while minimizing the possibility of iatrogenic damage (e.g., scuffing) to articular surfaces and structures (Fig. 3–11).

Joint lavage and irrigation of the operative field is provided by means of a port, or stopcock, on the sheath assembly. Extension tubing can be attached to the port to deliver fluids to the arthroscopic field. Outflow can be attained by using a 15-gauge 1½-inch needle, a butterfly needle, or a Teflon intravenous catheter. Other outflow devices with larger diameters are available that allow access to instruments. These outflow cannulas provide a locking mechanism for trochars and a outflow port on their side for irrigant flow.

All the necessary equipment for TMJ arthroscopy must be arranged in a convenient manner for efficient use in the operating room. The equipment must be positioned to accommodate cables, electrical cords, suction tubing, and anesthesia circuit tubing for optimal access and ease of use. Placement of the video monitor toward the head of the patient allows both the surgeon and the assistant a satisfactory view. The anesthesiologist should be away from the patient's head, out of the way. The nasoendotracheal tube should be secured to the head and longer extension tubes used in the anesthesia circuit to accommodate the distance to the anesthesia machine. The surgeon operates from the same side as the TMJ to be arthroscoped, while the assistant surgeon stands on the opposite side. Figure 3–12 shows the placement of all operating room equipment and personnel.

Arthroscopic equipment (Fig. 3–13) is delicate, and care must be exercised in its maintenance. Sterilization of metal instruments such as trocars and cannulas can be accomplished by conventional high-pressure steam autoclaving. Arthroscopes should be routinely gas sterilized (ethylene oxide gas) since repeated high-pressure steam sterilization eventually leads to deterioration of the adhesive seals on the lens. Most video cameras and cables are sealed and can be soaked in a cold sterilizing solution but more commonly are "bagged" (enclosed in sterile plastic wrapping) to preserve sterility. Fiberoptic cables contain multiple strands of light-conducting fibers. Repeated careless sharp bending or coiling of the cable will result in fracturing of the fibers and loss of light conductivity. These cables may be gas sterilized or autoclaved, but like arthroscopes, they will deteriorate with repeated high-pressure autoclaving. To

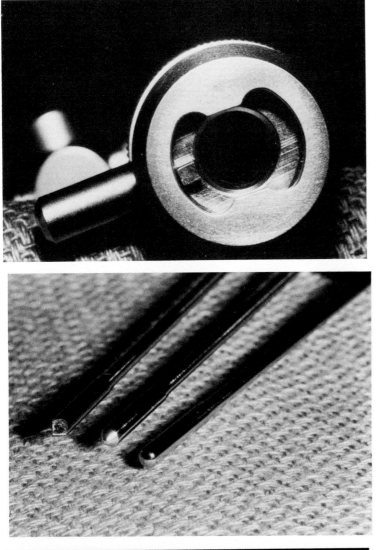

FIGURE 3–10   /   Self-locking mechanism
on canula.

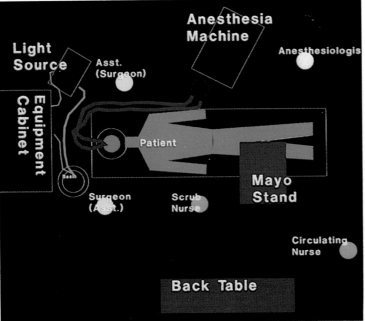

FIGURE 3–11   /   Trochars and
obturators. Left to right: sharp pyramidal
trochar, conical obturator, blunt
obturator.

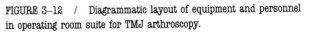

FIGURE 3–12   /   Diagrammatic layout of equipment and personnel
in operating room suite for TMJ arthroscopy.

FIGURE 3–12 cont'd   /   Equipment List

Mayo Stand
10-cc aspirating syringe—local anesthetic with vasoconstrictor
10-cc aspirating syringe—fluid for joint distension (e.g., lactated ringers, normal saline)
Inflow cannula
Trochars and obturators
　　　　　Blunt
　　　　　Pyramidal
　　　　　Sharp
Outflow cannula
15-gauge, 1½-inch spinal needle
Wolf 1.9-mm 5-degree arthroscope
Wolf 1.9-mm 20-degree arthroscope
Outflow tubing (IV extension tube)
Inflow tubing (IV extension tube)
Marking pen
20-cc syringe for joint lavage and irrigation

Head of Table
Basin—light cable, video camera
Light source
Cabinet—high-resolution video monitor
　　　　　video tape recorder
　　　　　video camera control unit

Back Table

Suction tubing
Drapes
Lap sponges
4 × 4 sponges
Cotton balls
Video camera bag
Towels for draping
Cotton tip applicators
1000-cc. graduated flask for irrigation fluid

Mosquito hemostats
Head dressing bandage
　　Two 4″ Kerlix gauze rolls
　　6″ bias cut stockinette
　　Round Band-aids
Celestone (steroid) in 2-cc syringe
　　1½ inch 20-gauge needle
Surgical instrument packs for open
　　arthrotomy if needed

prevent damage, it is always wise to check the manufacturer's recommendation before subjecting expensive equipment to the rigors of any method of sterilization.

References

Johnson L: Diagnostic and Surgical Arthroscopy. St. Louis, CV Mosby, 1981.
Seliga C: Personal communication, 1987.
Sharriaree HL: O'Connor's Textbook of Arthroscopic Surgery. Philadelphia, J.B. Lippincott, 1984.
Wetterman LA: From endoscopy to arthroscopy, in O'Connor RL (ed): Arthroscopy. Philadelphia, J.B. Lippincott, 1977.

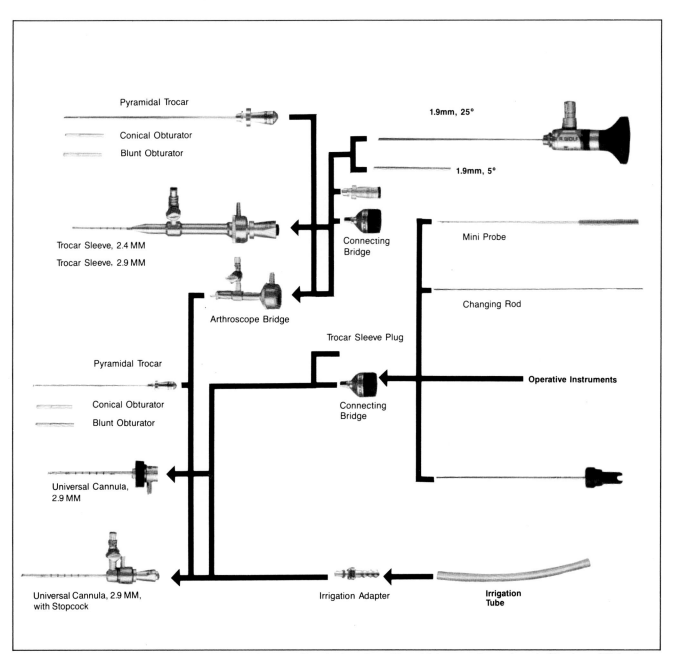

Pyramidal Trocar

Conical Obturator

Blunt Obturator

1.9mm, 25°

1.9mm, 5°

Trocar Sleeve, 2.4 MM

Trocar Sleeve, 2.9 MM

Connecting Bridge

Mini Probe

Arthroscope Bridge

Changing Rod

Trocar Sleeve Plug

Pyramidal Trocar

Conical Obturator

Blunt Obturator

Connecting Bridge

Operative Instruments

Universal Cannula, 2.9 MM

Universal Cannula, 2.9 MM, with Stopcock

Irrigation Adapter

Irrigation Tube

FIGURE 3–13 / Instrumentation for small joint arthroscopy. Note the interchangable and interconnective equipment. (Courtesy of Richard Wolf Medical Instrument Corp.)

4 Arthroscopic Technique

Part 1 / **Bruce Sanders**
Ralph D. Buoncristiani

Mandibular Manipulation and the Preauricular Depression

The arthroscopic technique begins with the assistant surgeon manipulating the mandible anteriorly and inferiorly. This maneuver allows some translation of the condyle out of the fossa and produces a palpable preauricular depression. This preauricular depression is a critical landmark for joint injection and arthroscopic entry. The surgeon may request that the assistant surgeon repeatedly relax and then activate the mandibular manipulation to define this depression. While the assistant surgeon manipulates the mandible and creates the preauricular depression, the surgeon constantly has his or her left index finger (if right-handed) in the depression (Fig. 4–1A-C).

Obese patients may not have palpable preauricular depressions. Effective low-risk TMJ arthroscopy may therefore be impossible and could be a contraindication for such patients.

FIGURE 4–1 / Mandibular manipulation and preauricular depression landmark. *A*, With the assistant surgeon manipulating the mandible downward and forward, the surgeon palpates the resultant preauricular depression overlying the right temporomandibular joint. *B*, Incorrect palpation of the preauricular depression because there is no manipulation of the mandible. *C*, The scrub nurse has a syringe of local anesthetic available for injection of the joint while the assistant surgeon manipulates the mandible and the surgeon palpates the preauricular depression.

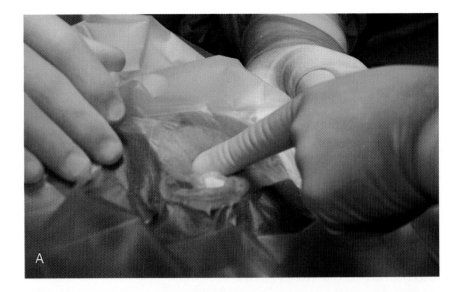

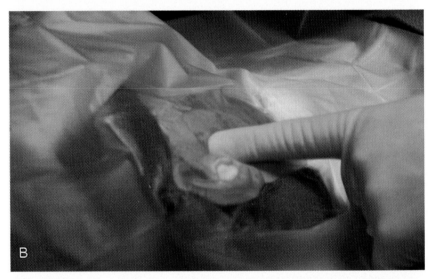

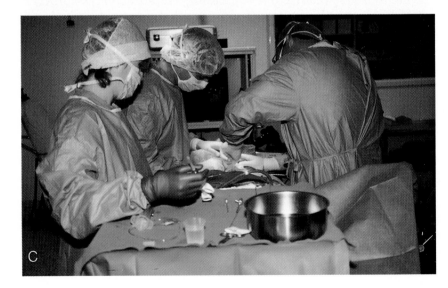

Joint Injection

Using a 20-gauge needle, the surgeon then injects the superior compartment with 1 to 2 ml of 0.5 percent lidocaine with 1:200,000 epinephrine. This is done for operative hemostasis and postoperative analgesia. Angulation of the needle puncture is from the inferolateral-posterior approach, so that the needle tip is aimed toward the posterior slope of the articular eminence. Next, 3 to 4 ml of lactated Ringer's solution is injected in a similar manner to distend the superior compartment. A backflow of fluid is seen, which confirms that the superior compartment has been adequately filled (Fig. 4–2A-E).

FIGURE 4–2 / Injection of the joint. *A*, With the mandible manipulated downward and forward by the assistant and the preauricular depression palpated, the superior compartment of the right TMJ is entered via an inferolateral-posterior approach, aiming the needle tip toward the posterior slope of the articular eminence. This technique greatly reduces the chance of puncture of the ear canal or glenoid fossa. *B*, Local anesthetic is slowly injected. The puncture technique is then repeated with a syringe of lactated Ringer's solution in order to distend the superior compartment of the TMJ. This technique makes puncture of the trochar easier and less traumatic to articular surfaces. Often the assistant will feel the mandible shifting downward and forward secondary to joint distention. *C* and *D*, Left TMJ manipulation, palpation of the preauricular depression, and joint injection via inferolateral-posterior approach. *E*, If aspiration produces blood into the syringe, the needle should be retracted and redirected or totally removed and the joint reinjected.

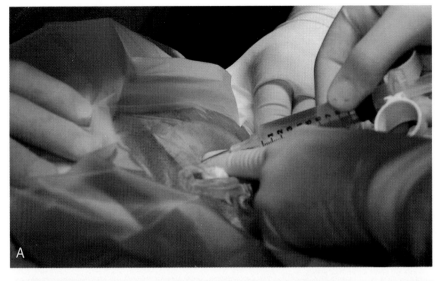

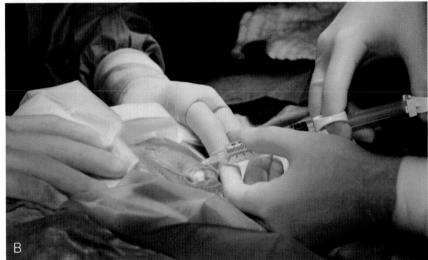

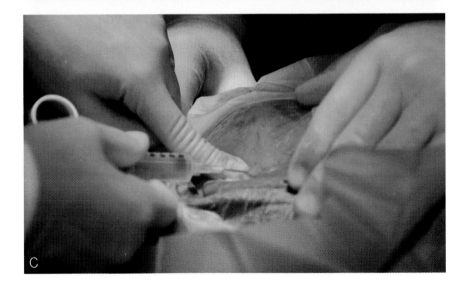

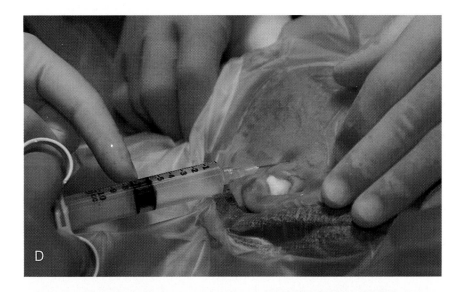

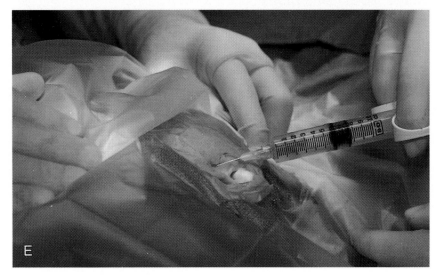

Puncture Technique

With mandibular manipulation and palpation of the preauricular depression still occurring, the superior compartment is punctured with a 1.9-mm pyramidal trochar in its sheath. Angulation is critical and, again, is from an inferolateral-posterior approach. As soon as the lateral temporomandibular capsule is punctured, the sharp trochar is replaced with the blunt, round obturator to avoid iatogenic "scuffing" of articular surfaces. Using the blunt obturator as a probe, the fossa and eminence are gently and carefully palpated for tactile orientation (Fig. 4–3A-E).

If the fossa and its contours, including the eminence, cannot be easily and readily palpated, the obturator and sheath should be withdrawn and the puncture procedure started again. Multiple repeated punctures are contraindicated and, if necessary, the procedures should be terminated.

Outflow Mechanism

Outflow is established by creating another portal approximately 3 to 5 mm anterior to the original portal. An outflow needle or a trochar with a sheath is used for puncture. The approach should be parallel to the original portal containing the blunt obturator and sheath. The outflow tubing is attached (Fig. 4–4A,B).

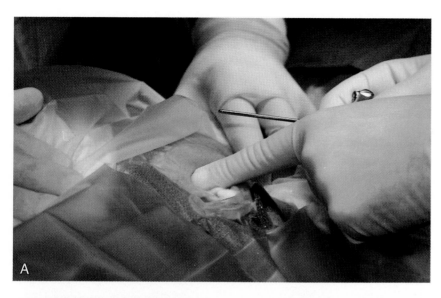

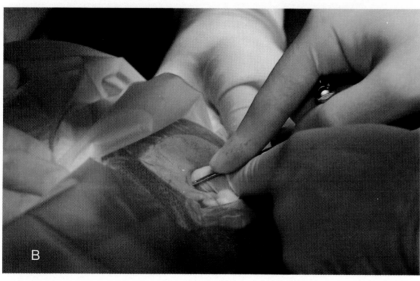

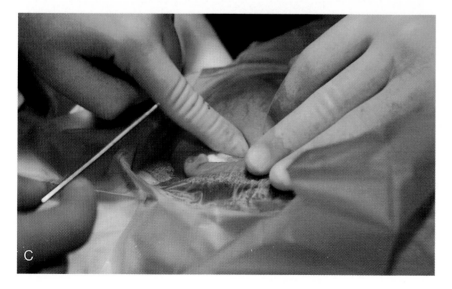

FIGURE 4–3 / Puncture technique. A and B, With mandibular manipulation and palpation of the preauricular depression of the right TMJ still active, puncture of the superior compartment lateral capsule is accomplished from the inferolateral-posterior approach. C and D, Left temporomandibular joint puncture. E, Gentle palpation of the fossa contour can be accomplished with the blunt obturator. (As soon as the capsule is punctured, the blunt obturator replaces the sharp trochar.)

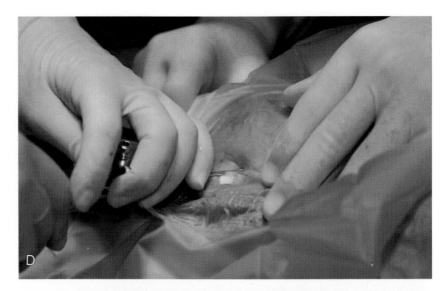

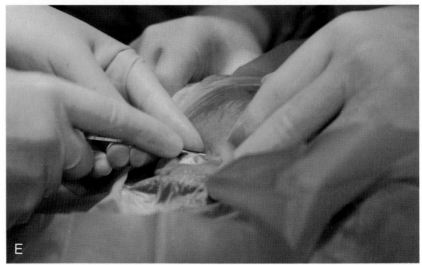

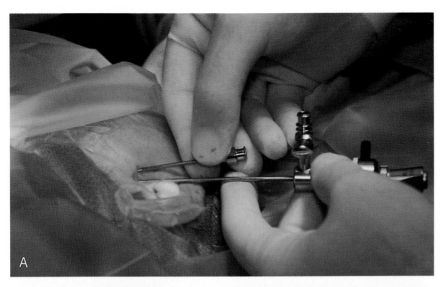

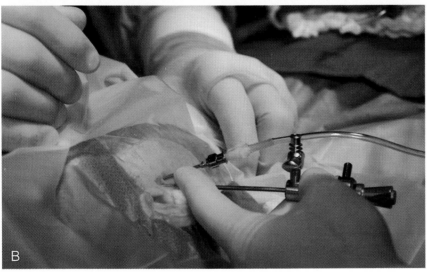

FIGURE 4–4 / Outflow mechanism. *A*, Outflow is established by placing a 15-gauge spinal needle anterior and parallel to the initial puncture. *B*, Outflow tubing is attached.

Arthroscope and VCR Camera, Inflow/Outflow Mechanism, and Monitor Viewing

The blunt obturator is removed from the sheath and the 1.9-mm arthroscope* with attached camera head is inserted. The inflow tubing is then attached to the sheath. One to 2 ml of lactated Ringer's solution is placed into the joint via the inflow to activate fluid escape through the outflow mechanism. A 20-ml or 50-ml syringe containing lactated Ringer's solution is attached to the inflow tubing as a source of irrigation. Once the inflow and outflow of irrigant have been established, arthroscopic examination of the TMJ may proceed (Fig. 4–5A-I).

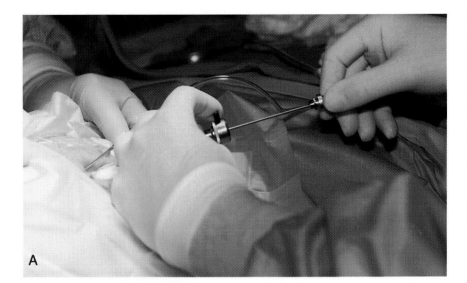

FIGURE 4–5 / Arthroscopy and VCR camera; inflow/outflow mechanism; monitor viewing. *A*, Blunt obturator is removed from sheath. *B*, Surgeon can reach the arthroscope and camera, which have been draped for sterility. (Many hospitals do not consider "soaking" the camera to be an acceptable sterile technique.) *C*, *D*, and *E*, Placement of the arthroscope and camera in sheath. Note the locking mechanism on the sheath. *F* and *G*, Scrub nurse slowly injects lactated Ringer's solution into inflow system, which activates outflow. *H*, Monitor viewing. *I*, Video recording is activated by pressing VCR button on camera.
Illustration continued on following page

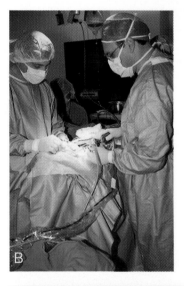

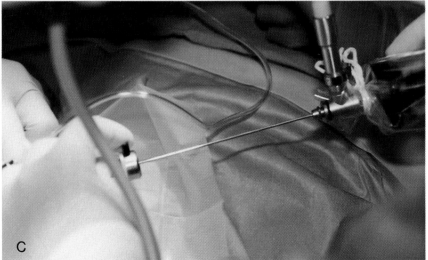

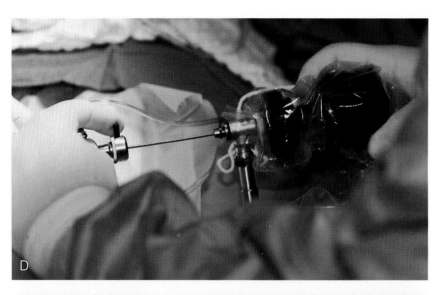

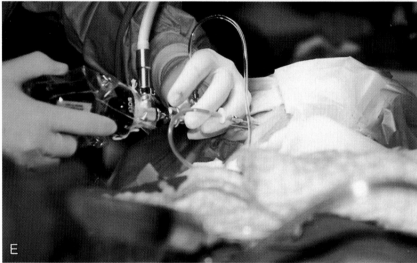

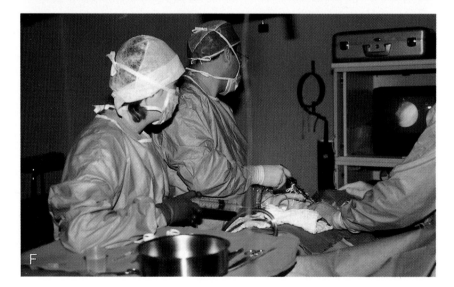

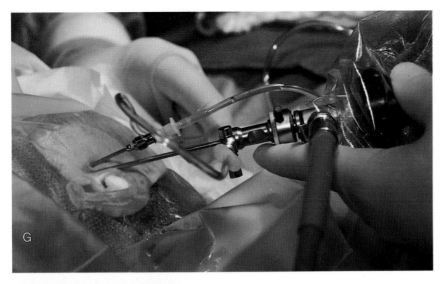

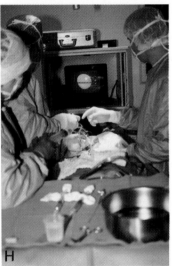

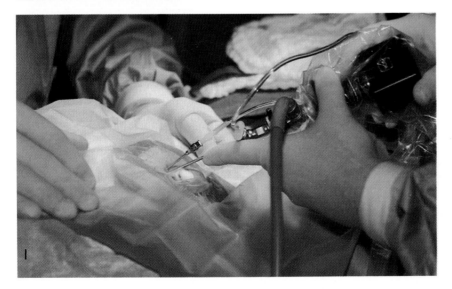

PART 2 / **Ken-Ichiro Murakami**

In 1975, Ohnishi reported the clinical application of arthroscopy by using a lateral puncture in the upper and lower joint cavities; this work was based on his fundamental study using dry skulls. Consecutive clinical arthroscopic examinations were described, complete with technical reviews (1982). Six different arthroscopic approaches to both upper and lower joint cavities were anatomically studied in human cadavers in 1981 (Murakami and Ito). Among these approaches, the inferolateral, posterolateral, and anterolateral punctures were applied to clinical arthroscopy (Murakami and Ito, 1984 and 1985). The endaural approach, used in combination with the lateral approach, was developed for the double-puncture technique (Ohnishi, 1982). Holmlund and Hellsing (1985) reported a TMJ arthroscopy study in which the average position or puncture point into the upper joint cavity (in cadavers) was 12 mm anterior to the tragus point and 2 mm below the tragus–lateral canthus line. The mean puncture depth was 27 mm. The safety of both arthroscopic puncture and examination was confirmed by using these techniques on fresh cadavers and then studying them by anatomical dissection (Westesson et al., 1986). Systematic arthroscopic examination by the inferolateral approach was reported to be a clinically useful arthroscopic technique in 1986 (Murakami and Ono). Triangulation for operative TMJ arthroscopy has been used recently by a few clinicians, who based their techniques on a study of cadavers (McCain, 1985).

The inferolateral approach and related arthroscopic techniques for clinical use are described below.

Equipment System

An Olympus Selfoscope system is shown in Figure 4–6. The diameter of each scope is 1.7 mm, and each outer sheath has a diameter of 2.0 mm. There are three different angles of view: straight, front-oblique, and 90-degree angled. Usually the front-oblique angle is used for obtaining wider fields of view (Fig. 4–7). The diameter of the scope is very fine: It has only a 39-degree visible field in water. Blunt and sharp trocars are necessary for penetrating into the joint cavity, and the punch is sometimes useful for biopsy and other procedures. A xenon light source (Olympus CLS-F) is a reliable cold light source for diagnostic and operative arthroscopy of the TMJ (Fig. 4–8).

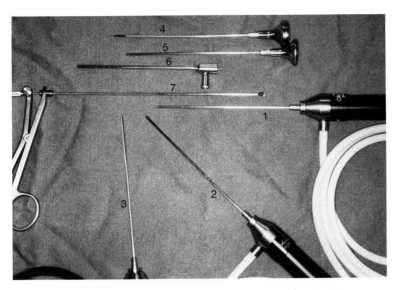

FIGURE 4–6 / Olympus Selfoscope system. Arthroscopes: *1*, straight view; *2*, front-oblique view; *3*, 90° angled view; *4*, sharp-tip trocar; *5*, blunt-tip trocar; *6*, outer sheath; *7*, punch.

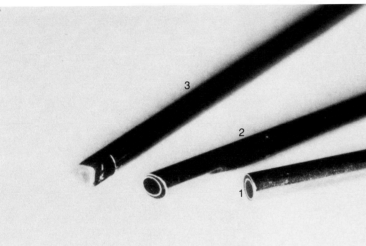

FIGURE 4–7 / Three kinds of Selfoscopes (1.7 mm diameter): *1*, straight view; *2*, front-oblique view; *3*, 90° angled view.

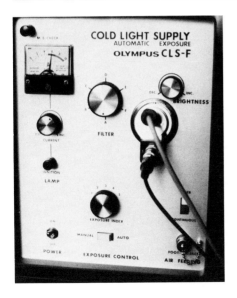

FIGURE 4–8 / Xenon light source, Olympus CLS-F. Flashlight is synchronized with 35-mm photograph.

Preparation and Anesthesia

Diagnostic arthroscopy is performed in the outpatient operating room. The patient sits in a dental chair and is given only local anesthesia. General anesthesia is indicated for patients undergoing surgical arthroscopy, and a supine position may be used, if necessary. All procedures are carried out under usual aseptic technique, and local anesthetic or normal saline solution for intra-articular use is injected. When local anesthesia is applied, an infiltration anesthetic with 0.5 percent lidocaine, including epinephrine, is injected first at the entry point (Fig. 4–9). Then, through a 21-gauge needle, 2 to 4 ml of a 2 percent lidocaine solution or normal saline is slowly injected into the upper joint cavity with a pumping procedure, which distends the articular capsule. For the lower joint cavity, 1.5 to 3 ml is used. This local anesthetic provides about one hour of anesthesia and makes the arthroscopic puncture easy and safe.

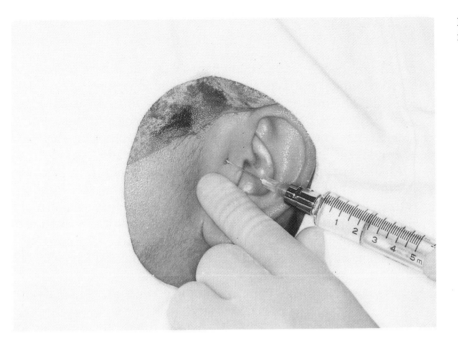

FIGURE 4–9 / Anesthetic is injected in
front of the tragus at the entry point.

The Inferolateral Approach

When the jaw opens, a skin pouch can be palpated at the retro-condylar area under the mandibular fossa and in front of the tragus. This pouch is the insertion point. Usually this point is found along the line of the tragus and lateral canthus. To avoid the superficial temporal artery, the angle of penetration should be such that the lateral rim of the mandibular fossa is pointed medially and slightly anteriorly. After the skin is punctured with a sharply tipped trocar, a blunt-tip trocar is inserted. Penetration of the superior articular cavity is accomplished at a depth of about 3 cm (Fig. 4–10). It is important to feel the temporal articular surface with the tip of the blunt trocar once the articular capsule is punctured. To enter the inferior articular cavity, the trocar is directed along the posterior surface of the mandibular condyle. After it touches the dorsal surface of the condylar head, the tip of the trocar is inserted into the lower posterior pouch along the condylar surface.

After the joint cavity is successfully punctured, the blunt trocar is replaced by the arthroscope, and observation is maintained under suitable pressure of normal saline extending the joint space (Fig. 4–11).

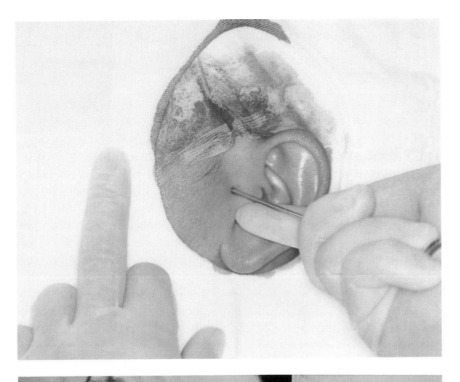

FIGURE 4–10 / Blunt-tip trocar with an outer sheath is inserted into the upper joint cavity. The operator's left finger points at about lateral canthus.

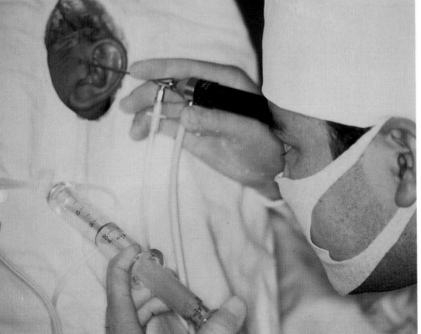

FIGURE 4–11 / Diagnostic arthroscopy examination under local anesthesia, single-puncture technique. The assistant surgeon maintains suitable extension of the joint capsule by injecting saline into the cavity.

Arthroscopic Maneuver and Visible Fields

At the beginning of systematic arthroscopic observation of the superior articular cavity, it is recommended that the upper posterior synovial pouch be visualized first (Fig. 4–12A). The synovial membrane, usually located at the bottom of the arthroscopic view, is an important anatomical landmark (Fig. 4–13A-B). For purposes of anatomical orientation, it is helpful to follow the synovium posteriorly as it reflects upward to the mandibular fossa. The synovial membrane appears soft. When the jaw is open, the synovial membrane stretches anteroposteriorly, because of the positional change of the articular disk. Normally, it is possible to see the articular disk sliding under the posterior surface of the articular eminence.

The next step in the examination is to move the arthroscope forward to the upper anterior synovial pouch (Fig. 4–12B). While the patient's jaw is open, the tip of the blunt trocar is put on the posterior slope of the articular eminence facing the disk, and while the jaw is closed, the trocar is slipped forward into the anterior recess. The synovial membrane on the anterior aspect of the disk and on the medial capsule are visible (Fig. 4–13C). The arthroscope is then pulled back to the first position as careful examination is made of the intermediate spaces (Fig. 4–12C), the articular eminence, and the articular surface of the disk (Fig. 4–13D). If the patient is under general anesthesia, the assistant surgeon can perform appropriate manipulation of the jaw in order to facilitate movement of the arthroscope for visualizing these structures.

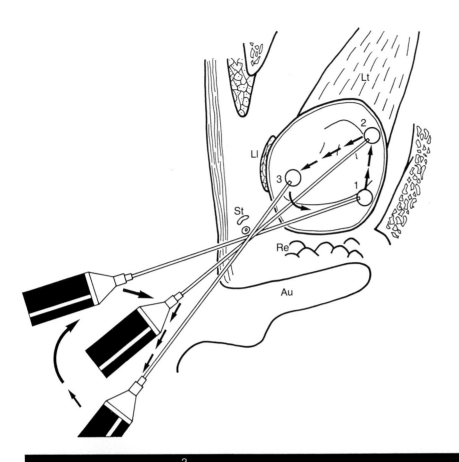

FIGURE 4–12 / Arthroscopic manipulation in the joint cavity. The drawing indicates the upper joint cavity viewed from above. The order is as follows: 1, upper posterior synovial pouch; 2, anterior synovial recess; 3, intermediate space, and return to the initial position. Lt, lateral pterygoid; Ll, lateral ligament; St, superficial temporal vessels; Re, retrodiskal pad; Au, auditory canal. (From Murakami K, Ono T: Temporomandibular joint arthroscopy by inferolateral approach. Int J Oral Maxillofac Surg 15:410–417, 1986.)

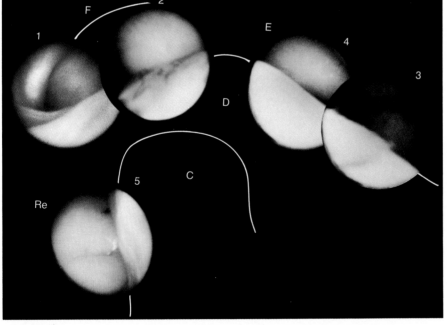

FIGURE 4–13 / Arthroscopic features of the normal temporomandibular joint. 1, upper posterior synovial pouch; 2, transitional area to the intermediate space; 3, upper anterior synovial recess; 4, intermediate space; 5, lower posterior synovial pouch. F, mandibular fossa; E, articular eminence (tubercle); D, articular disk; C, condylar head of the mandible; Re, retrodiskal pad.

When the arthroscope is inserted into the lower joint space, as described above, the visible field in the lower posterior pouch is limited because it is a narrower space than the one in the superior joint cavity (Fig. 4–14). To visualize the lower anterior recess, another puncture, such as by the anterolateral approach, should be made. Anatomical landmarks in the lower posterior pouch are the posterior surface of the mandibular condyle and the synovial membrane lining the retrodiskal pad (Fig. 4–13E). These two structures face each other. The surface view of the synovial membrane changes little regardless of the position of the jaw. Anatomical views of both upper and lower joint compartments (from above) and of the visible fields obtained by this approach are shown in Figure 4–15.

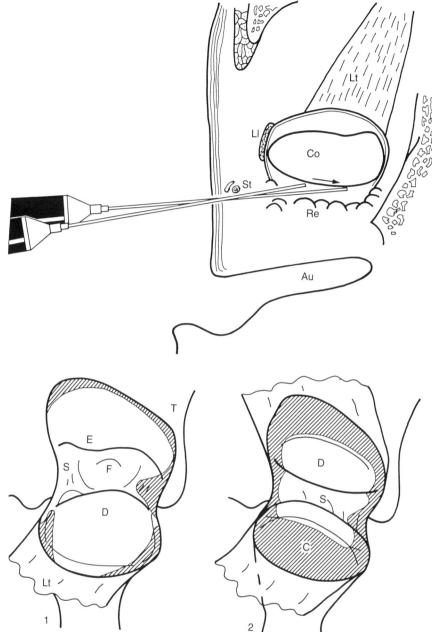

FIGURE 4–14 / Arthroscopic examination of the lower joint cavity viewed from above. (See Figure 4–12 for abbreviations.) The observation is limited to the lower posterior pouch. (From Murakami K, Ono T: Temporomandibular joint arthroscopy by inferolateral approach. Int J Oral Maxillofac Surg 15: 410–417, 1986.)

FIGURE 4–15 / Arthroscopic fields visualized by the inferolateral approach. Dark area is difficult to observe. The upper joint cavity (1) and the lower joint cavity (2) are opened from the back. T, temporal component; E, articular eminence; F, mandibular fossa; D, articular disk; Lt, lateral pterygoid, C, condyle head; S, synovial membrane. (From Murakami K, Ono, T: Temporomandibular joint arthroscopy by inferolateral approach. Int J Oral Maxillofac Surg 15:410–417, 1986.)

Documentation

Still photographs are easily taken with a 35-mm (Fig. 4–16) or 16-mm camera. Highly sensitive film, such as Kodak EL, is suitable for good color representation. Xenon light sources are better than tungsten ones. Video tape recording is highly recommended for both operative and educational purposes. Recently, several kinds of compact microvideo cameras have been made available for this purpose (Fig. 4–17).

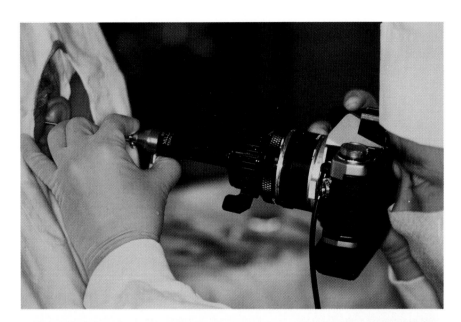

FIGURE 4–16 / Photograph obtained by 35-mm camera attached to the Selfoscope.

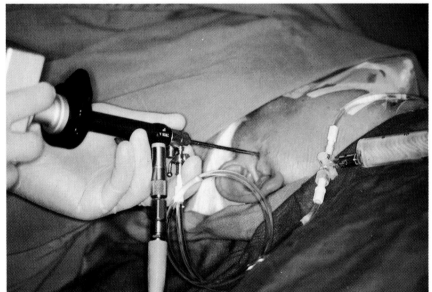

FIGURE 4–17 / Microvideo camera documentation with Storz 2.7-mm Needlescope.

References

Holmlund A, Hellsing G: Arthroscopy of the temporomandibular joint. An autopsy study. Int J Oral Surg 14:169–175, 1985.

McCain JP: Arthroscopy of the human temporomandibular joint. Abstracts, American Association of Oral and Maxillofacial Surgeons, Washington, D.C., 1985 Annual Scientific Session.

Murakami K, Ito K: Arthroscopy of the temporomandibular joint: Arthroscopic anatomy and arthroscopic approaches in the human cadaver. Arthroscopy 6:1–13, 1981 (in Japanese, abstract in English).

Murakami K, Ito K: Arthroscopy of the temporomandibular joint. Third report; Clinical experiences. Arthroscopy 9:49–59, 1984 (in Japanese, abstract in English).

Murakami K, Ito K: Arthroscopy of the temporomandibular joint, in Watanabe M (ed): Arthroscopy of Small Joints. Tokyo and New York, Igaku-Shoin, 1985, pp 128–139.

Murakami K, Ono T: Temporomandibular joint arthroscopy by the inferolateral approach. Int J Oral Maxillofac Surg 15:410–417, 1986.

Ohnishi M: Arthroscopy of the temporomandibular joint. J Stomatol Soc Jpn 42:207–213, 1975.

Ohnishi M: Development of arthroscopy of the temporomandibular joint and its clinical application. Bull Tokyo Med Dent Univ 31:478–512, 1982.

Westesson P-L, Eriksson L, Liedberg J: The risk of damage to facial nerve, superficial temporal vessels, disk, and articular surfaces during arthroscopic examination of the temporomandibular joint. Oral Surg 62:124–127, 1986.

5 Diagnostic Arthroscopy /
Ken-Ichiro Murakami

Arthroscopic pathological findings in the TMJ were first reported by Ohnishi in 1975, and his cumulative study was described in 1980. Arthroscopic observations were later done in patients with suppurative arthritis (Murakami et al., 1984) and suspected disk derangement (Hellsing et al., 1984). An autopsy study for evaluating the diagnostic accuracy of TMJ arthroscopy revealed that 100 percent of arthrotic changes and approximately 57 percent of remodeling changes could be detected (Holmlund and Hellsing, 1985). Arthroscopic differential diagnoses in patients with limited jaw opening disclosed three arthroscopic pathological groups: those with mild to moderate arthritis associated with the synovitis; those with arthrosis involving fibrosis and adhesion; and those with internal derangement and disk displacement (Murakami et al., 1986). Recently, Liedberg and Westesson (1986) studied the diagnostic accuracy of arthroscopic diagnosis in the upper compartment by using fresh cadavers, and they concluded that TMJ arthroscopy is highly specific but of low sensitivity.

Of importance is how to use this technique in conjunction with other diagnostic methods. Direct arthroscopic inspection of pathological change within the TMJ component is most reliable, and such findings are very useful for choosing therapeutic procedures.

Pathological Arthroscopic Findings

The synovial membrane responds to inflammation in the TMJ, and these changes can easily be detected arthroscopically in the synovial pouch. For instance, congestion, hyperemia, and microbleeding on the synovial membrane and mild to severe synovitis can be seen (Fig. 5–1). Synovial hyperplasia is occasionally detected in patients with rheumatoid arthritis (Fig. 5–2).

The arthroscopic features of fibrous changes initially appear as fibrillation or adhesion on the articular surfaces (Fig. 5–3). In advanced cases, the fibrous changes involve all inner joint surfaces and consist of fibrosis of the articular capsule and arthrosis (Fig. 5–4); cartilaginous changes are detected initially as chondromalacia (Fig. 5–5). Mild to moderate remodeling of the articular cartilage on the mandibular condyle and articular eminence are found in association with surface irregularity (Fig. 5–6).

Abnormality of the articular disk can be divided into two categories: disk malposition, followed by deviation in form (Fig. 5–7, left), and surface changes such as fibrillation, adhesion, and perforation (Fig. 5–7, right).

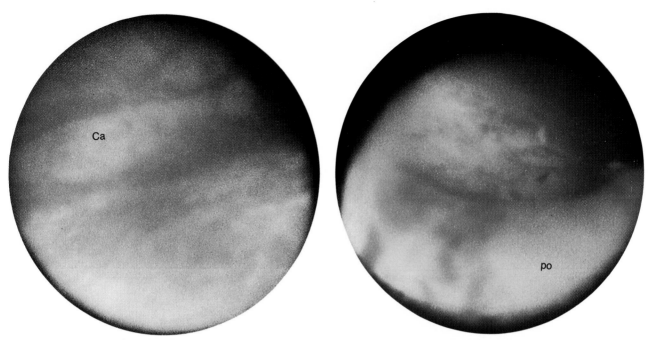

FIGURE 5–1 / Synovitis in the anterior synovial recess (*left*) in a patient with traumatic arthritis, and in the posterior synovial pouch (*right*) in a patient with closed lock. Dilatation of capillaries and reddened synovial membrane are observed on the inner capsular wall (Ca) and on the posterior discal attachment (Po).

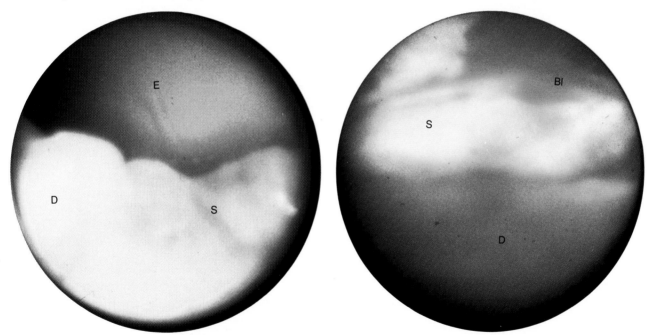

FIGURE 5–2 / Synovial hyperplasia in patients with rheumatoid arthritis. Right picture indicates a more active phase of rheumatoid arthritis with synovial proliferation. E, articular eminence; S, synovial membrane; D, articular disk; Bl, intra-articular bleeding. (From Murakami K, Ito K: Arthroscopy of the temporomandibular joint (3rd report). Clinical experiences. Arthroscopy 9:49–59, 1984.)

FIGURE 5–3 / Mild to moderate fibrosis is detected on the articular disk (*left*), and in the intermediate space (*right*). The former appears as surface adhesion, and the latter as clinically fibrous adhesion. D, articular disk; E, articular eminence.

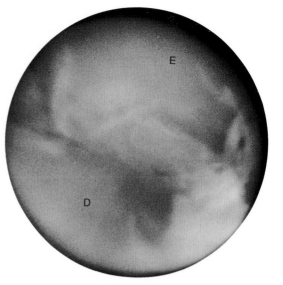

FIGURE 5–4 / Fibrosis of articular capsule (*left*) and arthrosis involving arthrotic changes on the articular eminence (*right*). E, articular eminence.

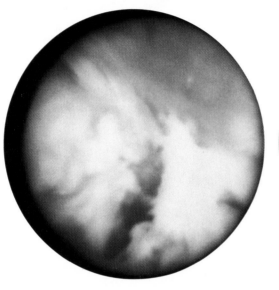

FIGURE 5–5 / Chondromalacia is detected on the articular eminence (*arrow*). E, articular eminence; Ca, anteromedial capsule in the upper anterior synovial recess; D, articular disk.

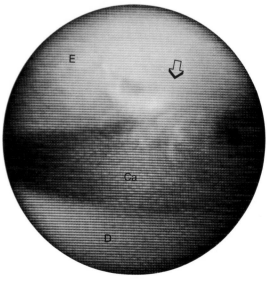

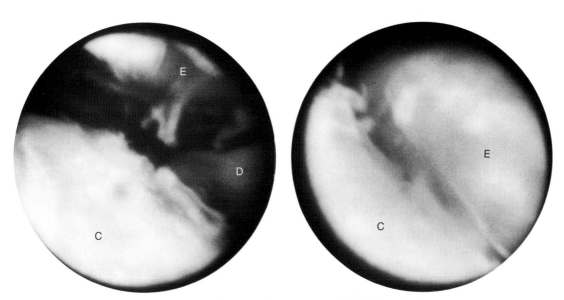

FIGURE 5–6 / Remodeling of the condyle and temporal component associated with arthrotic change. E, articular eminence; C, condylar head; D, ruptured disk.

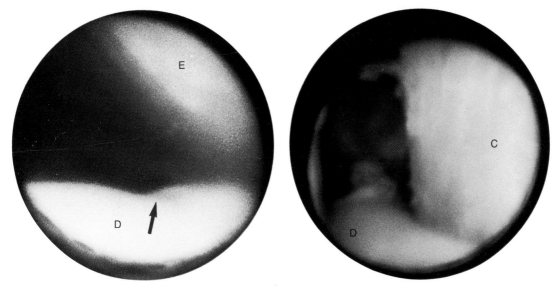

FIGURE 5–7 / Deviation (*left*) in form of the articular disk (*arrow*) and complete rupturing of the disk (*right*). E, articular eminence; D, articular disk; C, mandibular condyle with ruptured disk (D).

Diagnostic Group

Arthritis

Figure 5–8 shows the results of subacute traumatic arthritis in a 28-year-old man. Marked hyperemia, congestion, and microbleeding on the synovial membrane are seen in both the posterior synovial pouch and the anterior recess. In addition, the capillary network protrudes into the articular surface of the disk, which should normally be avascular. The patient had been suffering from dull pain of the TMJ that gradually began six months before the examination. Irrigation with normal saline and placement of steroids were effective for his symptoms.

Severe and chronic traumatic arthritis in a 37-year-old female is seen in Figure 5–9. This woman suffered violent pain from the restricted mobility in her right TMJ after a traffic accident six months earlier. Before arthroscopy, 2 ml of effusion was aspirated by joint puncture. The synovial membrane was swollen, hyperemic, and partially fibrotic. Irrigation and steroid placement were not helpful for this patient; the inflammation was so highly advanced that the lesion was suspected to be in an irreducible stage.

A case of suppurative arthritis is illustrated in Figure 5–10. Puncture prior to arthroscopy yielded yellowish-white pus. The synovial membrane was seen arthroscopically as severely reddened and swollen, and bleeding necrotic tissue was observed. Irrigation with antibiotic solution after saline washing was effective in treating the lesion.

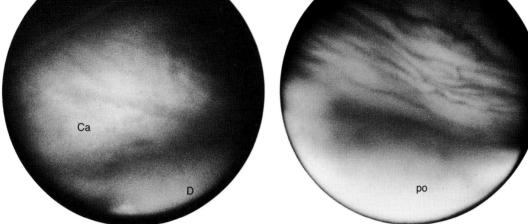

FIGURE 5–8 / Traumatic arthritis of the left TMJ in a 28-year-old man. Both the upper anterior synovial recess (*left*) and the upper posterior synovial pouch (*right*) show inflammatory signs. An abundant capillary network is present, but no abnormal disk position is detected. Ca, anteromedial capsular inner wall; D, articular disk; Po, posterior discal attachment.

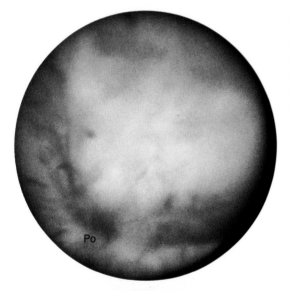

FIGURE 5–9 / Chronic traumatic arthritis of the right TMJ in a 37-year-old woman. Dilatation of the capillaries is observed through the swollen synovial membrane on the posterior discal attachment. Po, posterior discal attachment.

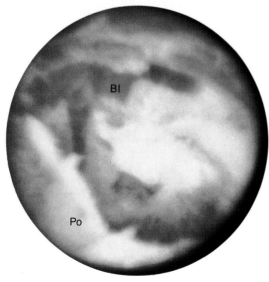

FIGURE 5–10 / Suppurative arthritis of the right TMJ in a 43-year-old man. A severely reddened and swollen synovial membrane is observed. Bleeding from the synovial structure is also seen. Po, posterior diskal attachment; Bl, bleeding and clots. (Redrawn from Murakami K, Matsumoto K, Iizuka T: Suppurative arthritis of the temporomandibular joint. J Maxillofac Surg 14:41–45, 1984.)

Internal Derangement

Figure 5–11 shows a 44-year-old female with chronic closed locking TMJ. Lower joint arthrography in the same patient clearly indicates anterior disk displacement without reduction and suggests severe malformation of the disk (Fig. 5–12). Arthroscopy did not reveal the whole joint structure, however. The following findings were obtained by the arthroscopy: stretching of the posterior attachment, obvious synovitis of the anterior aspect of the posterior attachment opposite the articular eminence, and fibrous change in the intermediate space. These features indicate that the disk was displaced anteriorly and did not reduce because of the fibrous adhesion at its anterior portion. Surgical findings in this case demonstrated that the articular disk was strongly displaced and deformed anteriorly, and the extensive intra-articular adhesion was observed in its anterior aspect (Fig. 5–13).

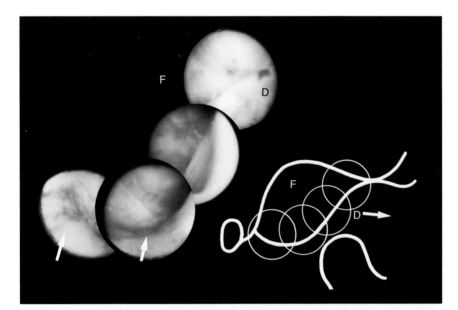

FIGURE 5-11 / Arthroscopic photographs showing a case of right TMJ internal derangement with persistent closed lock in a 41-year-old woman. The inset illustrates a schematic drawing of the visible area. The posterior diskal attachment is severely stretched anteroposteriorly, and marked synovitis with capillary dilatation (*arrows*) is seen. Fibrous adhesion is found in the intermediate space. F, mandibular fossa; D, articular disk.

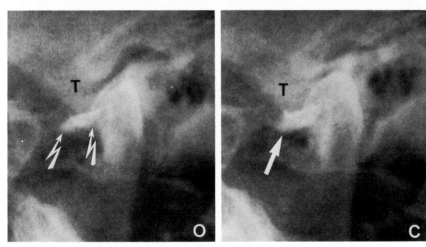

FIGURE 5-12 / Lower joint arthrography in the same patient as in Figure 5-11. Right picture indicates jaw in closed position, and the left shows the open position. Radiopaque dye in front of the condyle (*arrows*) demonstrates a representative finding of irreducible anterior disk displacement. T, articular tubercle.

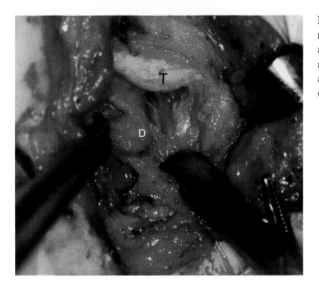

FIGURE 5-13 / Disk-repositioning surgery disclosed severely deformed and anteriorly displaced disk that adhered to surrounding structures. (Right is anterior.) T, articular tubercle; D, displaced articular disk.

A similar example of internal derangement in an 18-year-old man with chronic closed locking TMJ is shown in Figure 5–14. The posterior diskal attachment is severely stretched, and a dense fibrous articular disk appears deformed and displaced anteriorly. Synovitis is limitedly observed on the posterior diskal attachment, whereas no adhesion or perforation is detected. Lower joint arthrography reveals the typical features of anterior disk displacement without reduction (Fig. 5–15).

Arthrography is valuable for obtaining information about disk position, but it indicates few associated pathological conditions in TMJ internal derangement. On the other hand, arthroscopy provides pathological information on internal derangement of TMJ. The common valuable findings obtained by arthroscopy in patients with TMJ internal derangement are adhesion and disk perforation.

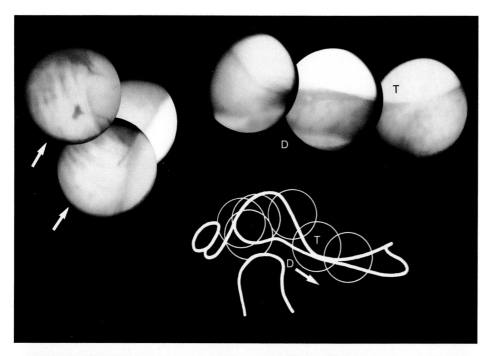

FIGURE 5–14 / An 18-year-old man with right TMJ closed lock. Arthroscopy demonstrates stretching of the posterior diskal attachment, displaced and deformed articular disk, and an increased upper anterior synovial recess. No fibrous change and less inflammatory change are observed on the inner surface of the upper joint cavity. T, articular eminence; D, articular disk.

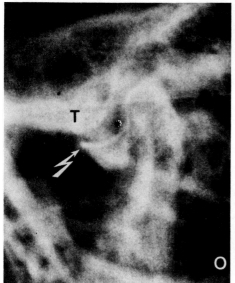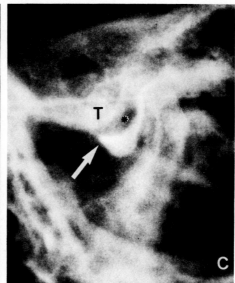

FIGURE 5–15 / Lower joint arthrography as in Figure 5–14. *Right*, jaw in closed position; *left*, jaw in open position. The diagnosis was irreducible anterior disk displacement with closed lock.

Adhesion

Figure 5–16 shows different stages of adhesion. Usually such adhesion is detected in the anterior aspect of the upper joint cavity, especially in the anterior recess. One hypothesis regarding adhesion in TMJ internal derangement is that the lesion progresses because of microbleeding following irreducible synovitis. Initial inflammation of the synovial membrane in the anterior recess appears to involve biomechanical stress associated with anterior disk displacement.

Perforation

Figures 5–17 and 5–18 show different types of perforation. The site of perforation in patients with anterior disk displacement is usually the posterior attachment or transitional zone to the articular disk. Rupture in the posterior diskal attachment is thought to result from its overstretching, caused by excessive anterior disk displacement.

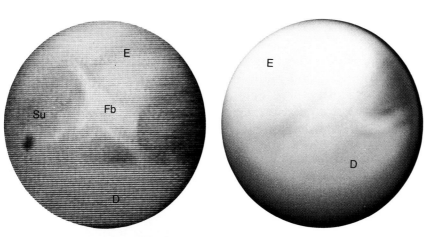

FIGURE 5-16 / Arthroscopic findings of intra-articular adhesion in patients with internal derangement with persistent closed lock. Left picture indicates right TMJ in a 34-year-old woman. Fibrous adhesion with synovitis in the upper anterior synovial recess is observed. Right picture shows surface adhesion at the intermediate space in the left TMJ in a 19-year-old woman. Extensive superficial fibrillation on the articular disk is seen. E, articular eminence; Fb, fibrous adhesion; Sv, synovitis; D, articular disk.

FIGURE 5-17 / Arthroscopic photograph of partial rupturing on the posterior diskal attachment in the right TMJ. The patient is a 35-year-old man. Arrows indicate ruptured tissues. F, mandibular fossa; Po, posterior diskal attachment.

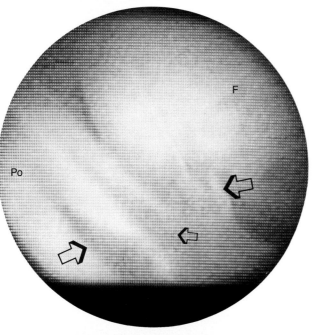

FIGURE 5-18 / Arthroscopy reveals the perforation of discal tissue in the right TMJ in a 35-year-old woman. Marked synovitis is associated with the perforated area (*long arrow*), in which the mandibular condyle protrudes into the upper joint cavity (*arrows*).

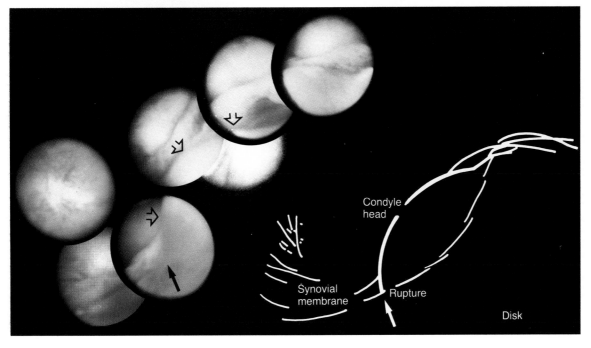

Arthrosis

It has been speculated that the initial phase of arthrosis involves fibrillation and fibrous adhesion. These pathological changes decrease the viscosity of articulation and represent a symptom of jaw hypomobility (Murakami et al., 1986).

Figure 5–19 presents a case of adhesion following trauma in a 68-year-old man. Despite efforts to open his jaw, the synovial membrane on the posterior attachment remained loose and dropped down. Since adhesion of the intermediate space was detected, lysis and ablation of the upper joint cavity were performed. Figure 5–20 shows the immediate postarthroscopic procedure. The fibrous adhesion was detected after surgical ablation, and smooth translation of the disk and stretching of the posterior attachment were obtained.

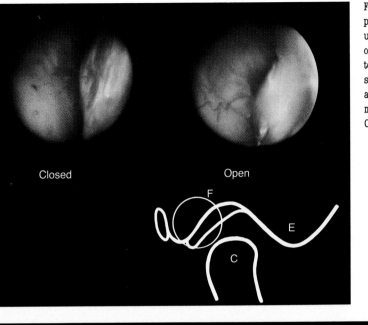

FIGURE 5-19 / Arthroscopic photographs demonstrate the view of the upper posterior synovial pouch in a case of adhesion after trauma. Despite efforts to open the jaw, neither disk sliding nor stretching of the posterior diskal attachment could be detected. F, mandibular fossa; E, articular eminence; C, condylar head of the mandible.

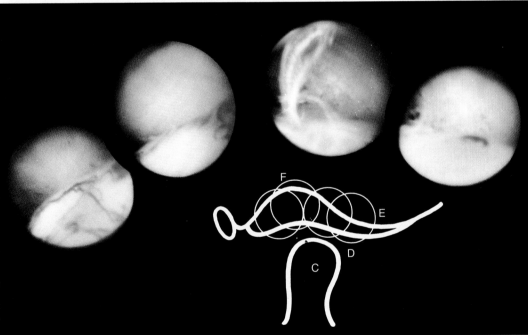

FIGURE 5-20 / Pictures indicate same example as in Figure 5-19 immediately after arthroscopic lysis and ablation. The articular disk could slide forward, and smooth stretching of the diskal attachment was seen. (See Figure 5-19 for abbreviations.) (From Murakami K et al: Diagnostic arthroscopy of the TMJ: Differential diagnoses in patients with limited jaw opening. J Craniomandib Pract 4:117-126, 1986.)

Figure 5–21 shows fibrosis of the articular capsule, or arthrosis, in a 41-year-old woman. Arthrography did not reveal positive findings, but arthroscopy disclosed extensive fibrous changes on all inner joint surfaces. No normal synovial membrane was detected, and arthrotic changes were seen on the temporal articular surface. The diagnosis, based on arthroscopy, was generalized fibrosis secondary to osteoarthrosis.

An advanced case, showing marked arthrosis with complete rupture of the disk, is seen in Figure 5–22.

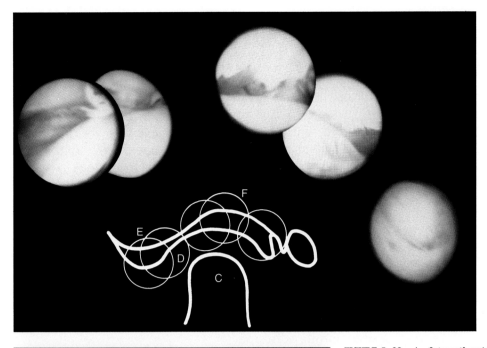

FIGURE 5-21 / Arthroscopic pictures indicate left TMJ with fibrosis of the articular capsule and arthrotic change in 41-year-old woman. Synovitis is not detectable. Extensive fibrillation is seen on the articular eminence. (See Figure 5-19 for abbreviations.)

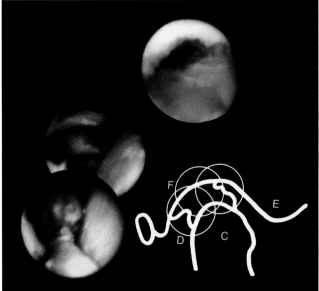

FIGURE 5-22 / Osteoarthrosis with complete ruptured disk in a 69-year-old man. (See Figure 5-19 for abbreviations.) (From Murakami K et al: Diagnostic arthroscopy of the TMJ: Differential diagnoses in patients with limited jaw opening. J Craniomandib Pract 4:117-126, 1986.)

TABLE 5-1
Clinical Cases Investigated with Arthroscopic Techniques

Patients	
Male	= 15
Female	= 27
Total	= 42
Age	
Range	= 14 to 69 years old
Mean	= 41.5 years
Joints	
Right	= 27
Left	= 12
Bilateral	= 6
Total	= 51

TABLE 5-2
Diseases Diagnosed Clinically Before Arthroscopy

DISEASE	NUMBER
Arthritis	10
Arthrosis	8
Internal derangement	21
Ankylosis	3
Other	5
Unknown	4

TABLE 5-3
Results of Arthroscopic Procedure

Diagnostic Results (n = 37)	
Diagnosed	= 28
Undiagnosed	= 1
Technical failure	= 8
Therapeutic Results (n = 14)	
Excellent	= 9
Good	= 2
Poor	= 3

Consecutive Cases

Between 1982 and 1985, 51 joints in 42 patients were examined (Table 5–1). Ages ranged from 14 to 69 years old, with a mean of 41.5 years. Classification of diseases is shown in Table 5–2: 10 cases of arthritis, including traumatic, rheumatoid, and suppurative; 8 cases of arthrosis, including fibrotic lesion, severe adhesion, and osteoarthrosis; 21 cases of internal derangement, involving 2 patients who reported clicking and 19 with closed lock (who included 4 cases of perforation and 3 of intra-articular severe adhesion). The four joints marked "unknown" were clinically difficult to diagnose. Joints in the other category included those with ankylosis and loose body.

The 51 joints undergoing TMJ arthroscopy could be divided into two groups: 37 diagnostic procedures and 14 therapeutic or operative arthroscopies. The therapeutic arthroscopies were performed for joint compartment irrigation, steroid placement for arthritis and synovitis, and joint débridement with lysis and ablation for intra-articular fibrous adhesion.

The results are shown in Table 5–3: there were 8 instances of technical failure among the 51 joints that were treated. Three of these patients had ankylosis, and five had pain that could not be controlled by local anesthesia.

In 28 cases in the diagnostic group, an accurate diagnosis could be made. In only one case was no useful information obtained by the arthroscopy.

Therapeutic results were poor in three cases, which consisted of one patient with traumatic arthritis who was not helped by joint irrigation and steroid placement and two patients with closed lock. These were later treated by open TMJ surgery.

Operative Management

Antibiotics were injected intravenously during the arthroscopic procedure and were continued by oral administration for three days. Common dressing was placed on the preauricular region, and a nonsteroidal anti-inflammatory agent was administered transorally. Steroids were injected into the joint cavity only in cases of obvious synovitis.

A stabilization splint was usually applied. The patients who underwent operative arthroscopy for joint adhesion and closed lock required physical exercise postoperatively.

Complications

No severe complications were encountered, but two mild side effects were seen: nausea and vomiting in reaction to the local anesthetic and a posterior disk attachment injury. The drug reaction subsided without severe consequences, and the disk repair was successfully done with a conventional disk-repositioning procedure.

Other complications of TMJ arthroscopy have been reported: facial nerve paralysis; extravasation of irrigation fluid; acoustic infection; intracapsular injury, including perforation to the middle cranial fossa; hemorrhage; broken instruments in the joint compartment; and postoperative infection. The incidence of those complications is, however, rare; J. McCain (1986) has reported an incidence rate of 1.7 percent.

Summary

For diagnostic purposes, arthroscopy is useful for obtaining additional information when routine arthrography fails to provide a diagnosis of intra-articular TMJ lesions. Arthroscopy also contributes valuable information about patients with internal derangement and helps in the detection of adhesion, synovitis, and pathological changes associated with perforations. When a surgeon is reviewing a surgical procedure such as disk repositioning, repair, or diskectomy, all available information is essential in each case. Arthroscopy should not be used, however, simply to confirm normal intra-articular joint conditions.

Arthroscopic treatment such as joint irrigation and steroid placement is indicated for mild to moderate synovitis. Operative arthroscopy is useful for patients with acute to subacute closed lock in whom lysis and ablation are used for associated adhesion. Occasionally, arthroscopic lysis and lavage may be indicated for arthrosis. Compared with open surgery, arthroscopy is a less traumatic procedure; however, its limitations should be considered in the treatment of each patient.

References

1. Hellsing G, Holmlund G, Nordenram A, Wredmark T: Arthroscopy of the temporomandibular joint. Examination of two patients with suspected disk derangement. Int J Oral Surg 13:69–74, 1984.
2. Holmlund A, Hellsing G: Arthroscopy of the temporomandibular joint. An autopsy study. Int J Oral Surg 14:169–175, 1985.
3. Westesson, P-L, Eriksson, L, Liedberg, J: The risk of damage to facial nerve, superficial temporal vessels, disk, and articular surfaces during arthroscopic examination of the temporomandibular joint. Oral Surg 62:124–127, 1986.
4. McCain, JP: Complications of arthroscopic surgery. Proceedings of the Symposium on TMJ Arthroscopy and Arthroscopic Surgery, Southern California Foundation of Oral and Maxillofacial Surgery, Long Beach, CA, 1986.
5. Murakami K, Matsuki M, Iizuka T, Ono T: Diagnostic arthroscopy of the temporomandibular joint. Differential diagnoses in patients with limited jaw opening. J Craniomandib Pract 4:118–123, 1986.
6. Murakami K, Matsumoto K, Iizuka T: Suppurative arthritis of the temporomandibular joint. Report of a case with special reference to arthroscopic observations. J Maxillofac Surg 15:41–45, 1984.
7. Ohnishi M: Arthroscopy of the temporomandibular joint. J Stomatol Soc Jpn 42:207–213, 1975 (in Japanese).
8. Ohnishi M: Clinical application of the arthroscopy in the temporomandibular joint diseases. Bull Tokyo Med Dent Univ 27:141–150, 1980.

6 Surgical Arthroscopy /
Bruce Sanders
Ralph D. Buoncristiani

The surgical arthroscopic procedure for persistent closed lock and for arthrosis is to sweep the superior compartment with a blunt probe to eliminate the suction cup effect of the disk to the fossa and to lyse adhesions (Sanders, 1986) (Sanders and Buoncristiani, 1987) (Fig. 6–1A–D). Thorough lavage, via the arthroscopic inflow and outflow mechanisms, is also carried out with lactated Ringer's solution (Fig. 6–2). Steroid medication is placed in the superior compartment if the tissue appears to be inflamed and hyperemic. Betamethasone (Celestone), 6 mg/ml, is employed, ¼ to ½ ml. Mandibular manipulation is also used to release closed lock with arthroscopic confirmation. Lysis and lavage is also a very helpful procedure in cases of arthrosis with adhesive capsulitis. No sutures are needed to close the wound (see Fig. 6–10). A small bandage is placed, and a full head dressing is applied. The patient receives intravenous antibiotics at the beginning of the procedure.

The pressure dressing is removed a few hours postoperatively, and ice is placed directly to the area. Jaw mobilization exercises are commenced the same day the patient is discharged from the outpatient hospital facility. Analgesics and antibiotics are prescribed. The patient is seen in the surgeon's office two to three days after surgery. Close cooperation with the patient's dentist and physical therapist is suggested for optimal rehabilitation. Long-term follow-up is recommended.

Complications of arthroscopy can include, but are not exclusive to, hemorrhage, infection, and damage to adjacent structures (middle cranial fossa; external, middle, or inner ear; blood vessels; nerves; and parotid gland). There may be no improvement in symptoms or worsening of symptoms. Contraindications to arthroscopic surgery include a nonpalpable preauricular depression, the presence of infection in the joint or ear, and the absence of clear indications of intracapsular temporomandibular joint pathology.

The surgeon must have extensive experience in open TMJ surgery and have the appropriate training in TMJ arthroscopic procedures before undertaking TMJ arthroscopy.

FIGURE 6–1 / A, Diagram of surface adhesions between the articular eminence and the disk. B, C, and D, Lysis of adhesions via superior compartment sweep. (B and C from Sanders B: Arthroscopic surgery of the temporomandibular joint. Oral Surg 62: 367, 1986.)

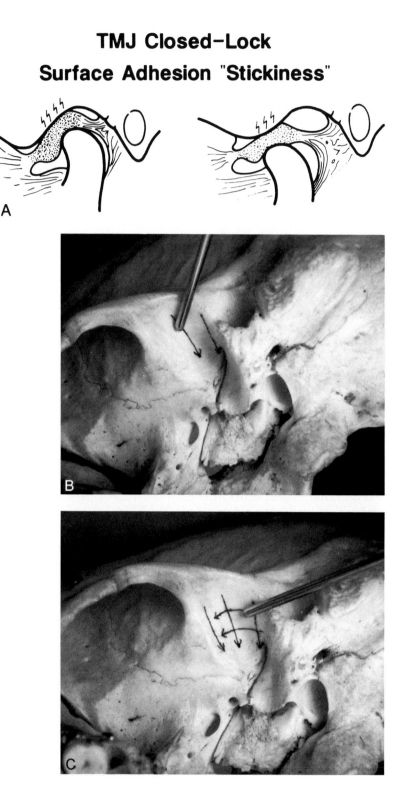

TMJ Closed–Lock
Surface Adhesion "Stickiness"

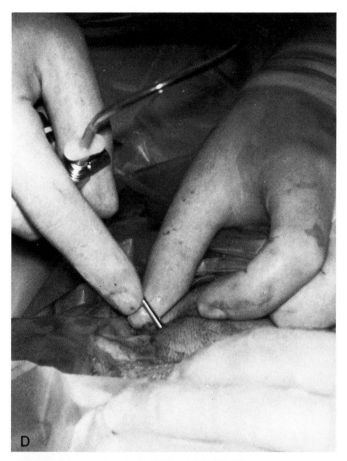

D

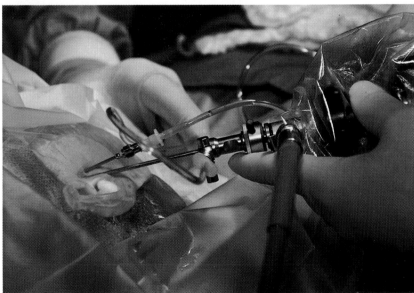

FIGURE 6–2 / Therapeutic lavage.

Clinical Experience

From 1985 to 1987, 137 TMJ arthroscopic diagnostic and surgical procedures were done in 92 patients. Forty-five patients had bilateral procedures, and 47 patients had unilateral procedures. Sixty-six (48.2 percent) right joints were done and 71 (51.8 percent) left joints. There were 86 female and 6 male patients, ranging in age from 11 to 57 years old, with a mean of 29 years (Table 6–1, Fig. 6–3). The preoperative diagnosis in these patients was either internal derangement with persistent closed lock or arthrosis with capsulitis.

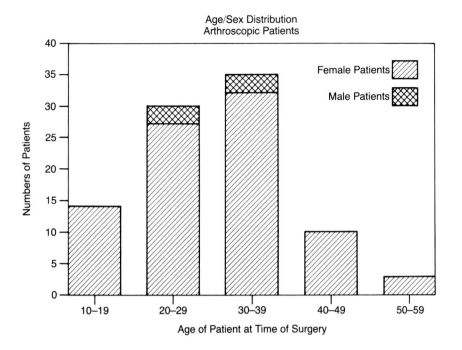

Age/Sex Distribution
Arthroscopic Patients

FIGURE 6–3 / Age and sex distribution of patients at time of surgery.

TABLE 6–1*
Arthroscopic Patient Data

PAT. INIT.	REC. NO.	DATE OF SURGERY	AGE	SEX	TMJ	DURATION OF SYMPTOMS YR.	MO.	CLINICAL DIAGNOSIS	RADIOGRAPHIC FINDINGS ON ARTH./TOMOGRAM	SIGNS AND SYMPT.	ARTH. SURG. DONE	ARTHROSCOPIC EXAMINATION FINDINGS	OPEN SUR. DONE	P.O. DUR. YR.	MO.	P.O. STAT.	COMPLICATIONS
LG	1	04/29/85	30	F	R	5	6	DJD	NRAD,MC	P,H	N	A,S,EF	Y	2	0	E	–0–
LG	2	04/29/85	30	F	L	2	0	DJD	NRAD	P,H	Y	S,A	N	2	0	E	–0–
BO	3	05/08/85	47	F	L	5	0	RA,DJD	DJD,P	P,H	N	P,DE,S,A	Y	1	11	E	–0–
BO	4	05/08/85	47	F	R	1	0	RA,DJD	DJD	P,H	Y	S,A	N	1	11	E	–0–
JM	5	05/22/85	18	F	R	7	0	RA,CL	NRAD,MC	CL,P	Y	S,A	N	1	11	E	–0–
JM	6	05/24/85	18	F	L	7	0	RA,CL	NRAD,MC	CL,P	Y	S,A	N	1	11	E	–0–
PS	7	05/28/85	39	F	L	6	0	DJD,C	DJD	P	N	S,A,P	Y	1	11	E	–0–
AH	8	06/03/85	49	F	L	1	0	DJD,CA	NRAD,DJD	P,H	N	A	Y	1	10	E	–0–
AH	9	06/03/85	49	F	L	1	0	DJD,CA	NRAD	P,H	Y	A,S	N	1	10	E	–0–
DE	10	06/17/85	28	F	R	8	0	RA	DJD	P,H	Y	A,S	N	1	10	F	–0–
DE	11	06/17/85	28	F	L	8	0	RA	DJD	P,H	N	DE,A,S	Y	1	10	F	–0–
SS	12	06/19/85	20	F	R	1	6	CL	NRAD	P,H	Y	A,DI	N	1	10	E	–0–
SS	13	06/19/85	20	F	L	1	6	CL	NRAD	P,H	Y	A,DI	N	1	10	E	–0–
ND	14	07/08/85	30	F	R	1	0	CL	NRAD	CL	Y	A,S	N	1	9	E	–0–
ND	15	07/08/85	30	F	L	1	0	CL	NRAD	P,CL	Y	A,S	N	1	9	E	–0–
MM	16	07/10/85	51	F	R	3	0	DJD	DJD	P,H	Y	A,S,EF	N	1	9	E	–0–
MM	17	07/10/85	51	F	L	3	0	DJD	DJD	P,IL	N	A,S,EF	Y	1	9	E	–0–

Table continued on following page

TABLE 6–1* *Continued*

Arthroscopic Patient Data

PAT. INIT.	REC. NO.	DATE OF SURGERY	AGE	SEX	TMJ	DURATION OF SYMPTOMS YR.	MO.	CLINICAL DIAGNOSIS	RADIOGRAPHIC FINDINGS ON ARTH./TOMOGRAM	SIGNS AND SYMPT.	ARTH. SURG. DONE	ARTHROSCOPIC EXAMINATION FINDINGS	OPEN SUR. DONE	P.O. DUR. YR.	MO.	P.O. STAT.	COMPLICATIONS
CD	18	07/22/85	19	F	L	2	0	CL	NRAD	P,CL	Y	A,S	N	1	9	E	–0–
GS	19	07/29/85	25	F	R	10	0	CA	DJD	P,H	N	FB	Y	1	9	E	–0–
GS	20	07/24/85	25	F	L	10	0	CA	DJD	P,H	N	FB	Y	1	9	E	–0–
CZ	21	08/06/85	24	F	R	2	0	CA	DJD	P	N	FB	Y	1	8	E	–0–
CZ	22	08/06/85	24	F	L	2	0	CA	DJD	P	N	FB	Y	1	8	E	–0–
JD	23	08/12/85	23	F	L	10	0	A	MC,DJD	H	Y	A	N	1	8	E	–0–
BG	24	08/13/85	11	F	L	0	4	CL	NRAD	CL	Y	A	N	1	8	E	–0–
MM	25	08/13/85	46	F	L	0	3	CL	RC,NRAD	CL	Y	A,S	N	1	8	E	–0–
DJ	26	08/27/85	35	M	R	2	0	CL	NRAD	P,H	Y	A	N	1	8	E	Severe ear infect.*
JD	27	08/19/85	37	F	R	0	3	CL	NRAD	P,H	Y	A,H	N	1	8	E	–0–
LM	28	08/19/85	19	F	R	0	3	CL	NRAD	CL	Y	A,S	N	1	8	E	–0–
LM	29	08/19/85	19	F	L	0	3	CL	NRAD	CL	Y	A	N	1	8	E	–0–
LO	30	08/21/85	25	F	L	1	0	DJD	DJD	P,H	N	FB	Y	1	8	G	–0–
KK	31	08/21/85	30	F	L	5	0	CA	DJD	P	N	FB	Y	1	8	G	–0–
KL	32	09/04/85	32	F	R	2	0	CA	NRAD	P	Y	A	N	1	7	E	–0–
KL	33	09/04/85	32	F	L	2	0	CA	NRAD	P	Y	A	N	1	7	E	–0–
TB	34	09/09/85	27	F	R	0	6	CA	DJD	P	Y	A,S	N	1	7	G	–0–
TB	35	09/09/85	27	F	L	0	6	CA	DJD	P	Y	A,S	N	1	7	G	–0–
SB	36	09/10/85	28	F	R	0	6	CA	DJD	P	N	–0–	Y	1	7	E	–0–
SB	37	09/10/85	28	F	L	0	6	CA	DJD	P	N	–0–	Y	1	7	E	–0–
EF	38	09/11/85	27	F	R	11	0	DJD,CA	P	P,IL	Y	P,DI,A	N	1	7	E	–0–
EF	39	09/11/85	27	F	L	11	0	DJD,CA	P	P,IL	Y	A,S	N	1	7	E	–0
TF	40	11/13/85	30	F	R	14	0	CL	NRAD,MC	CL	Y	A	N	1	5	G	–0–
TF	41	11/13/85	30	F	L	14	0	CL	NRAD	CL	Y	A	N	1	5	G	–0–
MH	42	12/09/85	21	M	R	1	0	CL	NRAD	CL	Y	A	N	1	4	E	–0–
MH	43	12/09/85	21	M	L	1	0	CL	NRAD	CL	Y	A	N	1	4	E	–0–
VF	44	12/09/85	31	F	L	0	6	CL	NRAD	CL	Y	A,H	N	1	4	P	–0–
VF	45	12/09/85	31	F	R	0	6	–0–	NRAD	CL	Y	A,DI	N	1	4	E	–0–
KN	46	01/06/86	22	F	R	1	6	DJD	DJD	P	Y	MC,A,EF	N	1	3	E	
KN	47	01/06/86	22	F	L	1	6	RA	DJD	P	Y	MC,A,EF,S	N	1	3	E	–0–
CA	48	01/06/86	18	F	R	2	6	CL	MC,NRAD	P,H	Y	DI,A	N	1	3	E	–0–
CA	49	01/16/86	18	F	L	2	6	CL	NRAD	P,H	Y	DI,A	N	1	3	E	–0–
LH	50	01/13/86	32	F	R	3	6	CL	NRAD,MC	P	Y	A	N	1	3	E	Mild ear infect.

TABLE 6-1* *Continued*

Arthroscopic Patient Data

PAT. INIT.	REC. NO.	DATE OF SURGERY	AGE	SEX	TMJ	DURATION OF SYMPTOMS YR.	MO.	CLINICAL DIAGNOSIS	RADIOGRAPHIC FINDINGS ON ARTH./TOMOGRAM	SIGNS AND SYMPT.	ARTH. SURG. DONE	ARTHROSCOPIC EXAMINATION FINDINGS	OPEN SUR. DONE	P.O. DUR. YR.	MO.	P.O. STAT.	COMPLICATIONS
LH	51	01/13/86	32	F	L	3	6	MPD,CL	NRAD	P	Y	A,MC	N	1	3	E	–0–
MM	52	12/13/85	29	F	R	1	0	CL	NRAD	P,H	Y	A,H,MC	N	1	4	E	–0–
MM	53	12/13/85	29	F	L	1	0	CL	NRAD	P,H	Y	A,H,MC	N	1	4	E	–0–
LT	54	01/20/86	30	F	R	3	0	DJD,MPD	DJD	P	N	MC,EF,DI,A,	Y	1	3	E	–0–
LT	55	01/20/86	30	F	L	3	0	MPD	MC	IL	Y	DI	N	1	3	E	–0–
RR	56	01/27/86	23	F	L	3	6	CL	NRAD	P	Y	A,S,MC	N	1	3	E	–0–
LB	57	02/03/86	17	F	L	0	4	CL	NRAD,P,MC	P,CL	Y	DI,A	N	1	2	E	–0–
LN	58	02/03/86	15	F	R	1	6	CL,CA	NRAD	P,CL	Y	DI,A	N	1	2	E	–0–
LN	59	02/03/86	15	F	L	1	6	CL,CA	NRAD	P,CL	Y	DI,A	N	1	2	G	–0–
EB	60	02/03/86	38	F	L	10	0	DJD	DJD	P,IL	Y	A,S	N	1	2	E	–0–
LB	61	02/17/86	36	M	R	0	2	CA,MPD	MC	P,H	Y	A,S	N	1	2	E	–0–
LB	62	02/17/86	36	M	L	0	2	CA,MPD	MC	P,H	Y	A,S	N	1	2	E	Mild ear infection
BS	63	03/03/86	41	F	R	2	0	CL,CA	NRAD	P,H	Y	A,MC,H	N	1	1	E	–0–
BS	64	03/03/86	41	F	L	2	0	CL,CA	NRAD	P,H	Y	A,MC	N	1	1	E	–0–
NB	65	03/10/86	23	F	L	0	1	CL	NRAD	P	Y	A,MC,H	N	1	1	E	–0–
RR	66	03/10/86	18	F	L	1	4	CL	NRAD	P,H	Y	A,MC	N	1	1	E	–0–
KB	67	03/31/86	18	F	R	0	4	CL,MPD	RAD	P	Y	A,MC	N	1	0	E	–0–
KB	68	03/31/86	18	F	L	0	4	CL,MPD	NRAD	P	Y	A,H	N	1	0	E	–0–
LA	69	03/31/86	44	F	R	0	4	CL	NRAD	P,H	Y	DI,A,H	N	1	0	G	–0–
PP	70	04/07/86	29	F	L	2	3	CL	NRAD,MC	P	N	DI,MC,A	Y	1	0	G	–0–
MK	71	04/07/86	43	F	R	1	0	CL,MPD	NRAD	P	Y	DI,MC,A	N	1	0	E	–0–
DN	72	04/21/86	30	F	R	10	0	RA	MC,NRAD,P	P	Y	MC,A,S,H	N	1	0	E	–0–
DN	73	04/21/86	30	F	L	10	0	RA	MC	P	Y	MC,A,S,H	N	1	0	E	–0–
ML	74	04/21/86	30	M	R	1	5	CL	MC	P,H	Y	A,MC	N	1	0	G	–0–
ML	75	04/21/86	30	M	L	1	5	CL	MC	P,H	Y	A,MC	N	1	0	G	–0–
PG	76	04/21/86	49	F	R	10	0	DJD	NRAD	P	Y	A,MC,DI,H	N	1	0	G	–0–
LM	77	04/28/86	30	F	R	1	3	DJD	DJD	P	Y	DI,A	N	1	0	G	–0–
LM	78	04/28/86	30	F	L	1	3	DJD	DJD	P,H	N	A,S	Y	1	0	G	–0–
TB	79	05/05/86	27	F	R	7	0	CA	H	P	Y	A,C,H	N	0	11	G	–0–
TB	80	05/05/86	27	F	L	7	0	CA	H	P	Y	A,MC,S,H	N	0	11	E	–0–
VJ	81	05/19/86	34	F	R	0	4	IL	MC,NRAD	P	N	DI,MC,A	Y	0	11	G	–0–
SB	82	05/19/86	31	F	R	2	–0	CL,CA	NRAD	P,H	N	A	Y	0	11	E	–0–
SB	83	05/19/86	31	F	L	2	0	CA	MC	P	N	A	Y	0	11	E	–0–

Table continued on following page

TABLE 6–1* *Continued*
Arthroscopic Patient Data

PAT. INIT.	REC. NO.	DATE OF SURGERY	AGE	SEX	TMJ	DURATION OF SYMPTOMS YR.	MO.	CLINICAL DIAGNOSIS	RADIOGRAPHIC FINDINGS ON ARTH./TOMOGRAM	SIGNS AND SYMPT.	ARTH. SURG. DONE	ARTHROSCOPIC EXAMINATION FINDINGS	OPEN SUR. DONE	P.O. DUR. YR.	MO.	P.O. STAT.	COMPLICATIONS
CS	84	06/02/86	29	F	L	7	0	MPD,DJD	NRAD,MC	P,H	Y	MC	N	0	10	E	–0–
MN	85	06/02/86	43	F	R	15	0	MPD,DJD	DJD	P	Y	S,MC	N	0	10	G	–0–
VS	86	06/17/86	30	F	R	1	7	DJD	MC,RC,P,NRAD	P,H	Y	DI,MC,A,H	N	0	10	G	–0–
VS	87	06/17/86	30	F	L	1	7	DJD	MC,RC,NRAD	P,H	Y	DI,MC,A,H	N	0	10	G	–0–
SD	88	06/17/86	45	F	R	3	6	DJD	MC,DJD	P,IL	Y	S,MC,DI,A	N	0	10	G	–0–
KK	89	06/30/86	17	F	R	0	6	CL	NRAD	P,H	Y	DI,A	N	0	9	E	–0–
LS	90	06/30/86	27	F	R	0	8	–0–	NRAD,MC	P	Y	DI,A	N	0	9	E	–0–
LH	91	07/07/86	22	M	R	0	–0	CL	NRAD	P	Y	DI,H	N	0	9	E	–0–
LH	92	07/07/86	22	M	L	0	0	CL	NRAD,P,MC	P,H	Y	DI,A	N	0	9	E	–0–
RL	93	07/07/86	38	F	L	0	11	CL	NRAD	P,H	Y	DI,A,S	N	0	9	E	–0–
LM	94	07/28/86	22	M	R	0	5	DJD	MC	P,H	Y	DI,A	N	0	9	E	–0–
LM	95	07/28/86	22	M	L	0	5	DJD	NRAD,MC	P,H	Y	DI,A	N	0	9	E	–0–
CL	96	08/09/86	36	F	R	6	0	CL	NRAD	P,H	Y	A,MC,H	N	0	8	E	–0–
CL	97	08/04/86	36	F	L	6	0	CL	NRAD	P,H	Y	A,MC	N	0	8	E	–0–
PM	98	07/21/86	31	F	R	4	0	DJD	DJD	P,H	Y	A,MC,DI	N	0	9	E	–0–
CB	99	07/21/86	38	F	R	5	0	MPD,CL	NRAD	P	Y	DI,A,S	N	0	9	E	–0–
CB	100	08/11/86	32	F	L	0	10	CL	MC,NRAD	P,H	Y	A,S,MC	N	0	8	E	–0–
CM	101	08/11/86	23	F	L	0	8	CL	NRAD	P,H	Y	A,S,DI,MC	N	0	8	E	–0–
LF	102	08/11/86	25	F	L	0	2	CL	NRAD	P,H	Y	A	N	0	8	E	–0–
VB	103	08/18/86	17	F	R	4	–0	CL	NRAD,H	P,H	Y	A	N	0	8	E	–0–
CW	104	08/18/86	33	F	R	0	2	DJD	DJD	P	Y	A,MC,EF,S	N	0	8	E	–0–
CW	105	08/18/86	33	F	L	0	2	DJD	DJD	P	Y	A,MC,EF,S	N	0	8	E	–0–
JM	106	09/15/86	30	F	R	4	6	CL	MC	P,H	Y	A	N	0	7	E	–0–
JM	107	09/15/86	30	F	L	4	6	CL	NRAD,MC	P,H	Y	A,DI	N	0	7	E	–0–
TG	108	09/15/86	25	F	L	5	0	CL	NRAD,MC	P,IL	Y	Y	N	0	7	E	–0–
SW	109	09/21/86	31	F	R	1	6	CL	NRAD	P	Y	A,DI	N	0	7	E	–0–
SW	110	09/21/86	31	F	L	1	6	CL	RAD	P	Y	A,DI	N	0	7	E	–0–
MD	111	09/29/86	20	F	L	0	2	CL	NRAD	P,H	Y	MC,CI,A,H	N	0	6	G	–0–
LC	112	09/29/86	36	F	R	0	3	DJD	DJD	P	N	MC,A	Y	0	6	G	–0–
LC	113	09/29/86	36	F	L	0	3	DJD	DJD	P	Y	A,MC,DE	N	0	6	G	–0–
JL	114	10/16/86	21	F	L	0	10	CL	DJD	P,H	Y	MC,A,S	N	0	6	P	–0–
SY	115	10/20/86	35	F	R	7	0	RA	DJD	P,H	Y	A,MC,S,H	N	0	6	E	–0–
SY	116	10/20/86	35	F	L	7	0	RA	DJD	P,H	Y	A,MC,S,H	N	0	6	E	–0–
GH	117	10/20/86	32	F	R	0	10	CL	NRAD,MC	P,H	Y	A,EF,DI,H	N	0	6	E	–0–

TABLE 6–1* *Continued*
Arthroscopic Patient Data

PAT. INIT.	REC. NO.	DATE OF SURGERY	AGE	SEX	TMJ	DURATION OF SYMPTOMS		CLINICAL DIAGNOSIS	RADIOGRAPHIC FINDINGS ON ARTH./TOMOGRAM	SIGNS AND SYMPT.	ARTH. SURG. DONE	ARTHROSCOPIC EXAMINATION FINDINGS	OPEN SUR. DONE	P.O. DUR.		P.O. STAT.	COMPLICATIONS
						YR.	MO.							YR.	MO.		
LH	118	10/20/86	23	F	R	1	0	DJD,MPD	NRAD,P	P,H	Y	MC,A,H	N	0	6	E	–0–
LH	119	10/20/86	23	F	L	1	0	DJD,MPD	RAD	P,H	Y	MC,A,H	N	0	6	E	–0–
MP	120	11/03/86	20	F	R	0	7	CL	NRAD	P,H	Y	A,H,DI	N	0	5	E	–0–
JL	121	11/03/86	19	F	L	1	0	CL	NRAD,MC	P,H	Y	DI,A,MC	N	0	5	E	–0–
LB	122	11/10/86	18	F	R	5	0	CL	NRAD,MC	P,H	Y	DI,H,MC	N	0	5	E	–0–
NM	123	11/10/86	56	F	R	0	6	DJD	NRAD,P,MC	P,H	N	P,S,EF	Y	0	5	E	–0–
ES	124	12/15/86	41	F	L	1	6	CA,CL	NRAD,H	P,H	Y	A,MC,H,S	N	0	4	E	–0–
DW	125	12/12/86	32	F	R	3	9	CA	DJD	P,H	Y	A,MC	N	0	4	G	–0–
GG	126	12/12/86	32	F	R	16	0	CL,MPD	NRAD	P,H	Y	DI,MC,A	N	0	4	E	–0–
LW	127	01/12/87	37	F	R	0	7	MPD,CA	MC	P,H	Y	DI,EF,H,A	N	0	3	E	–0–
LW	128	01/12/87	37	F	L	0	7	MPD,CA	RAD,MC	P,H	Y	DI,EF,H,A	N	0	3	E	–0–
LG	129	01/26/87	17	F	R	12	0	CL,DJD	DJD	P,H	Y	MC,A,DI,H	N	0	3	P	–0–
LG	130	01/26/87	17	F	L	12	0	CL,DJD	DJD	P	Y	MC,A,DI,H	N	0	3	P	–0–
MM	131	01/12/87	24	F	R	1	0	CL	DJD	P,H	Y	MC,DI	N	0	3	E	–0–
SM	132	01/12/87	26	F	L	2	6	DJD,MPD	NRAD	P,H	Y	A,H,MC	N	0	3	E	–0–
AG	133	01/26/87	38	F	R	0	9	CL	MC,H	P	Y	MC,DI,A	N	0	3	E	–0–
AG	134	02/02/87	33	F	R	0	5	CL	NRAD	P,H	Y	DI,A	N	0	2	E	–0–
HT	135	02/23/87	27	F	R	0	8	CL	NRAD,MC	P,H	Y	A	N	0	2	E	–0–
HT	136	02/23/87	27	F	L	0	8	CL	NRAD,MC	P,H	Y	A	N	0	2	E	–0–
BG	137	02/23/87	57	F	L	0	6	CL	DJD,RC	P,H	Y	DI,A,S,MC	N	0	2	E	–0–

KEY TO ABBREVIATIONS: Clinical diagnosis: DJD = degenerative joint disease; CL = closed lock; RA = rheumatoid arthritis; A = ankylosis; MPD = myofascial pain dysfunction. Radiographic Findings on Arthrogram/Tomogram: NRAD = nonreducing anteriorly displaced disk; DJD = degenerative joint disease; MC = morphologic changes; P = perforation of disk; H = hypomobility of condyle; RC = retropositioned condyle; RAD = reducing anteriorly displaced disk. Signs and Symptoms: P = pain; H = hypomobility; CL = closed lock. Arthroscopic Examination Findings: A = adhesions; MC = morphologic changes; DI = displaced disk; H = hyperemia, increased vascularity; S = synovitis; DE = destroyed disk; EF = eburnation of fossa; FB = fibrous barrier intact; P = perforation. Postoperative Status: E = excellent; G = good; P = poor. IL = intermittent lock. *Resultant hearing defect.

*From Sanders B, Buoncristiani R: Diagnostic and surgical arthroscopy of the temporomandibular joint:Clinical experience with 137 procedures over a 2-year period. J Craniomandib Disord 1:202–213, 1987.

The etiology of the persistent closed lock cases was determined to be macro-trauma or multiple instances of micro-trauma to the affected temporomandibular joints. Preoperative arthrography was used in most cases when the tomographic appearance was relatively normal. Arthroscopic findings for the closed lock patients included surface adhesions (sticking of the superior surface of the disk to the anterior portion of the fossa and articular eminence), fibrillations of articular surfaces (Fig. 6–4A and B), superior compartment adhesions (Fig. 6–5A-D), an anteriorly displaced disk without reduction (Fig. 6–6), and morphologic and inflammatory changes in the disk and synovial lining (Fig. 6–7).

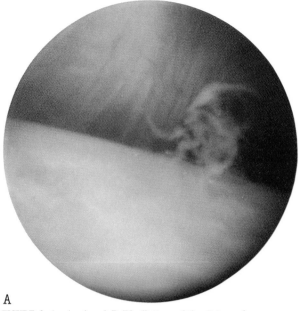

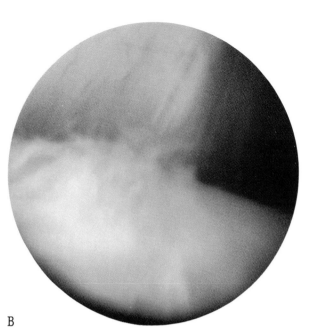

A

B

FIGURE 6–4 / *A* and *B*, Fibrillations of the disk surface.

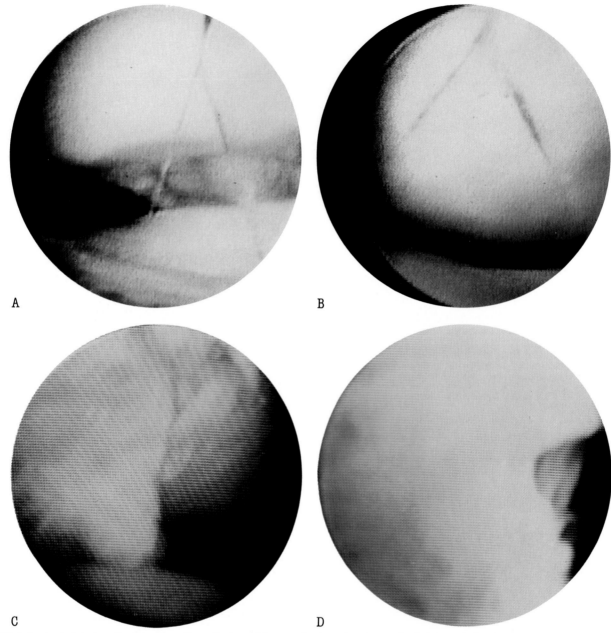

A

B

C

D

FIGURE 6–5 / *A*, Anterior adhesions; *B*, position adhesions; *C*, heavy adhesions at eminence; *D*, almost a complete fusion of disk to fossa with very heavy adhesions. (*D* from Sanders B: Arthroscopic surgery of the temporomandibular joint. Oral Surg 62:367, 1986.)

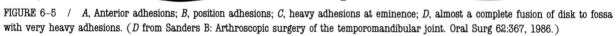

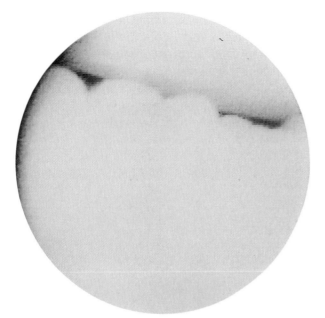

FIGURE 6–6 / Gross stretching and loosening of posterior
attachment, indicating chronic anteriorly displaced disk.

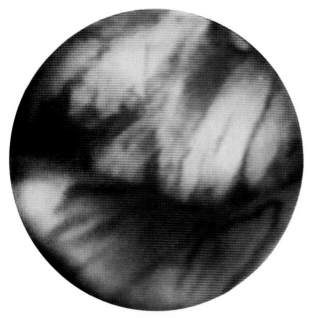

FIGURE 6–7 / Hyperemia of posterior attachment and synovial
lining status posttrauma and acute closed lock. (From Sanders B:
Arthroscopic surgery of the temporomandibular joint. Oral Surg 62:
367, 1986.)

A total 101 of the arthroscopic procedures had the preoperative diagnosis of persistent closed lock and 36 had the diagnosis of arthrosis with capsulitis. Of the 137 arthroscopic procedures, 115 were surgical (therapeutic) arthroscopies. Twenty-two of the 137 arthroscopies were diagnostic only, which resulted in immediate arthrotomy (Fig. 6–8). Arthroplasty, meniscectomy, and Silastic fossa implant was the treatment in all of the arthrotomy cases (Table 6–2).

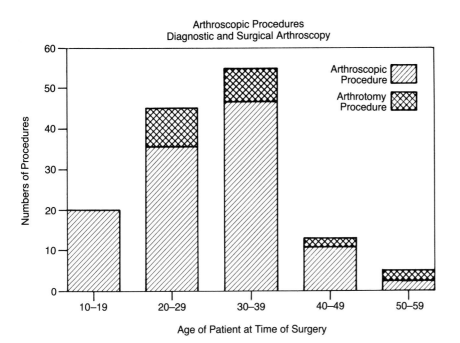

FIGURE 6–8 / Summary of arthroscopic (diagonal slope down to the left) and arthrotomy (diagonal slope down to the right) procedures, distributed by age of the patient.

TABLE 6–2
Summary of Patient Data

AGE	MALE	FEMALE	AVERAGE DURATION OF SYMPTOMS		NO. OPEN PROCEDURES	NO. CLOSED PROCEDURES
			Years	Months		
10 to 19	0	14	2 yr. &	6 mo.	0	20
20 to 29	3	27	2 yr. &	5 mo.	9	36
30 to 39	3	32	3 yr. &	1 mo.	9	46
40 to 49	0	10	4 yr. &	4 mo.	2	11
50 to 59	0	3	1 yr. &	0 mo.	2	2
Totals	6	86	2 yr. &	11 mo.	22	115

Results have been generally successful (Fig. 6–9). The more acute the closed lock, the more asymptomatic the patient postoperatively. Long-term chronic closed lock may have significant morphologic changes in the disk, and recapturing of the disk into a normal physiological position is not possible with lysis and lavage only (Fig. 6–10). The patient will achieve significant relief of symptoms, however, in most cases (Fig. 6–11A-G).

Determining the success or failure rate included evaluating subjective symptoms postoperatively along with objective findings. Ninety-four of 115 (82 percent) of the surgical arthroscopies were ranked as excellent result (little or no complaints and excellent jaw opening and function). Sixteen of the 115 (14 percent) of the surgical arthroscopies were ranked as good result (minimal or occasional moderate complaints and good jaw opening and function). Five of the 115 (4 percent) of the surgical arthroscopies were ranked as a poor result (moderate or severe complaints and poor jaw opening and function). Four of the five failures have undergone open TMJ surgery with meniscectomy and Silastic fossa implant. One case is scheduled for open surgery.

There were three complications, all of which were postoperative ear infections. Two were relatively minimal problems with full resolution of the otic problem and good temporomandibular joint result. One patient had a severe postoperative middle-ear infection that resulted in a significant hearing defect.

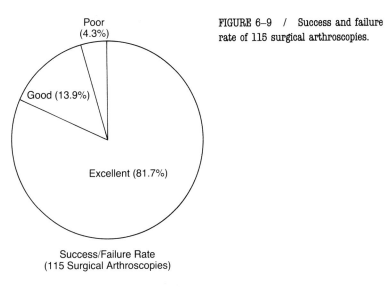

FIGURE 6–9 / Success and failure rate of 115 surgical arthroscopies.

Poor
(4.3%)

Good (13.9%)

Excellent (81.7%)

Success/Failure Rate
(115 Surgical Arthroscopies)

SUPERIOR COMPARTMENT ARTHROSCOPIC SWEEP

To Release Closed Lock

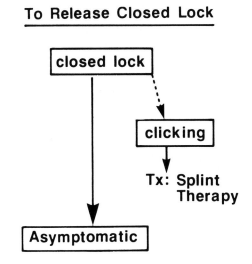

FIGURE 6–10 / After release of acute closed lock, the patient most likely will not have clicking. After release of very chronic closed lock, there may be clicking secondary to morphological changes in the disk. Splint therapy may be helpful to eliminate the clicking.

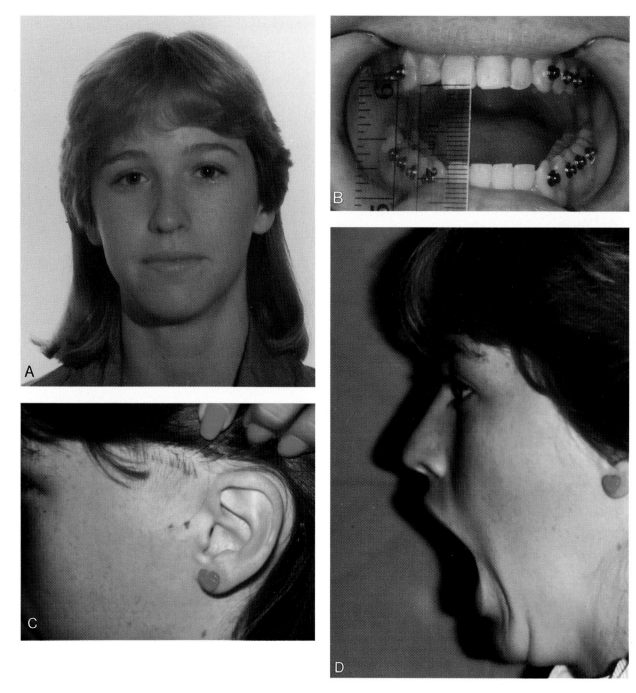

FIGURE 6–11 / A and B, Prearthroscopy closed lock of left TMJ. C
and D, One day postarthroscopy. Note the lack of sutures and full
oral opening.

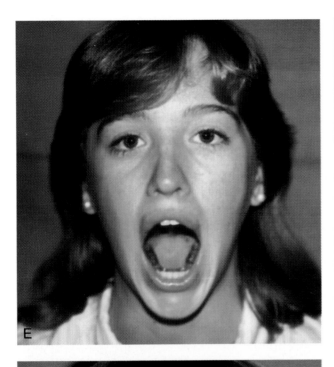

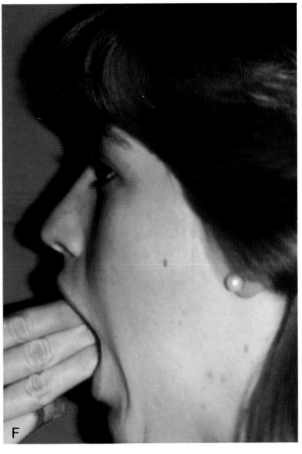

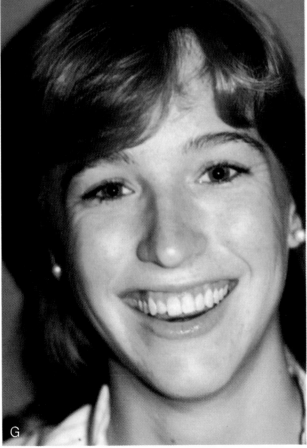

FIGURE 6–11 *Continued* / *E* and *F*, Note mandibular stabilizing splint and excellent opening. *G*, The patient is asymptomatic (picture taken two years postoperatively). (*C* and *D* from Sanders B: Arthroscopic surgery of the temporomandibular joint. Oral Surg 62: 367, 1986.)

Summary

Arthroscopy can be an important diagnostic and therapeutic modality in the treatment of some intracapsular TMJ disorders. Internal derangement with persistent closed lock and arthrosis with adhesive capsulitis are examples of problems for which arthroscopy can be used. Therapeutic (surgical) arthroscopy is an alternative to arthrotomy ("open" TMJ surgery) and can be very effective in eliminating symptoms of preauricular pain and mandibular hypomobility secondary to internal derangement with persistent closed lock (acute and chronic) and arthrosis with adhesive capsulitis when nonsurgical therapy has been unsuccessful.

Surgical arthroscopy has certain advantages over arthrotomy. It can be done as an outpatient procedure. It is a very brief operation; on the average it takes 10 to 30 minutes. No sutures are required. There is minimal swelling and minimal (to moderate) pain. For these reasons, jaw exercises can commence a few hours after surgery. Usually, full oral opening is obtained one to three days postoperatively. Patient acceptance and satisfaction are generally outstanding. If indicated, arthrotomy can be done immediately following arthroscopy or as a staged secondary procedure.

References

Sanders B: Arthroscopic surgery of the temporomandibular joint: Treatment of internal derangement with persistent closed lock. Oral Surg Oral Med Oral Pathol 62:361–372, 1986.

Sanders B, Buoncristiani, R: Diagnostic and surgical arthroscopy of the temporomandibular joint: Clinical experience with 137 procedures over a 2-year period. J Craniomandib Disord 1:202–213, 1987.

7 Analysis of Arthroscopically Treated TMJ Derangement and Locking /

Glenn T. Clark

David G. Moody

Bruce Sanders

Closed locking, or restricted translation of the condyle, involves condylar movement restriction due to disk perforation, disk deformation, disk–articular surface adhesion, disk displacement without reduction, or any combination of these conditions. Because the disk must rotate fully from an anterior position to a posterior position relative to the condyle in order to achieve full translation (Fig. 7–1A and B), any significant deformation, adhesion, or displacement without reduction produces this movement restriction. If the disk does not achieve its normal relationship with the condyle, fossa, and articular eminence during mandibular movement, a clear restriction of jaw opening, described as a "closed lock," will result (Fig. 7–2A and B). The preceding incoordination or clicking phase and the subsequent locking phase are not usually accompanied by any obvious radiographic osseous changes (Fig. 7–3).

The progression of this condition can eventually cause perforation of the disk and subsequent osseous remodeling of the condyle and temporal fossa in an adaptive attempt to restore normal movement. Arthroscopy has recently been advocated as a therapeutic procedure for the management of acute and sometimes chronic closed locking of the temporomandibular joint.[1–25] Because arthroscopy is a new procedure, it is necessary to provide the patient with a full disclosure of the following: (1) alternative treatments available; (2) results of no treatment; (3) potential complications of the proposed treatment; and (4) likelihood of success of the proposed treatment.

FIGURE 7–1 / Rotation of the disk as the condyle achieves full translation. *A*, closed position; *B*, wide-open position.

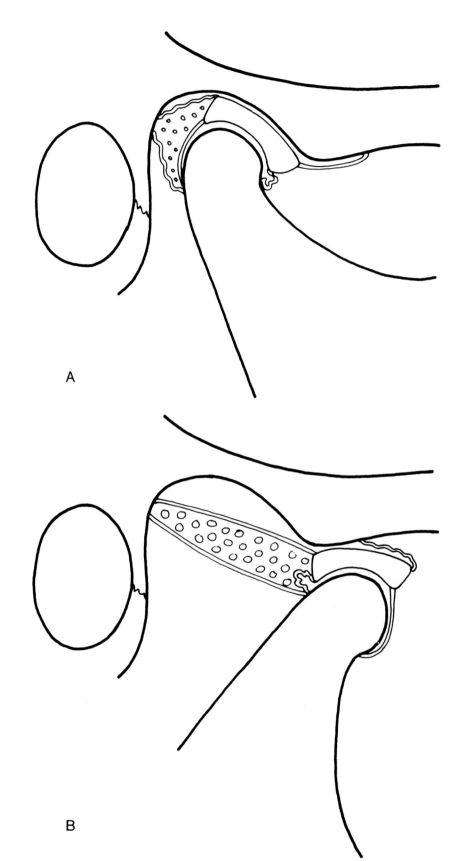

A

B

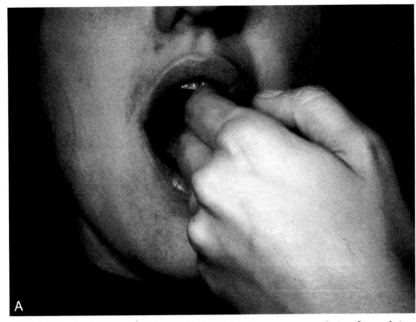

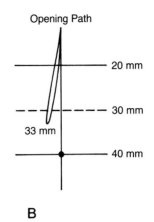

B

FIGURE 7-2 / A, Because of restricted translation, patient can get only two fingers between her teeth. B, Diagram showing the extent and path of opening of a patient with restricted translation of one condyle with slight deflection of the jaw to the side on opening.

FIGURE 7-3 / Radiograph (lateral tomogram) showing the typical appearance of a condyle with acute locking; there is no significant radiographic flattening, bony spurring, or decreased joint space.

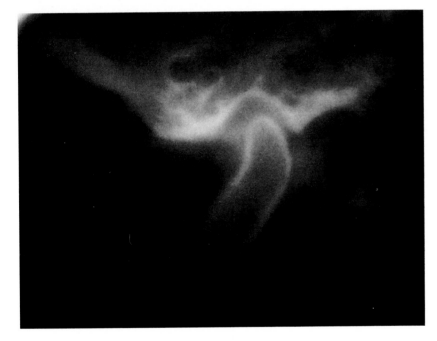

Although information exists in the literature regarding the prognosis for patients with TMJ closed lock without surgical treatment, little literature exists on the possible complications and prognosis for success of arthroscopic surgery of the TMJ.

This chapter is a preliminary report of data from six patients who had a diagnosis of acute or subacute closed locking confirmed by an arthrogram. Their evaluation involved an assessment of jaw movement ability, pain levels, and functional ability not only before surgery but also at four to eight weeks and at six months postoperatively. These patients all presented initially to the oral and maxillofacial surgeon with complaints of limited opening and preauricular pain.

All six patients received bilateral axially corrected sagittal tomograms of their temporomandibular joints, and these radiographs were evaluated for abnormalities. The patients also underwent upper and lower joint space arthrography of the involved joint preoperatively (Fig. 7–4A and B). During the arthrographic procedure, tomograms were taken to document the findings, which were interpreted by a dentist-arthrographer.

Arthroscopic Procedure

The procedures performed on these patients involved placement of the arthroscope in the superior compartment of the temporomandibular joint. This compartment was then flushed with a physiological saline or Lactated Ringer's solution, and arthroscopic probes were used to release any adherence between the disk and the articular surface.

An attempt was made to probe and visualize as much of the superior compartment as possible. No significant disk or attachment perforations were noted during arthroscopic visualization.

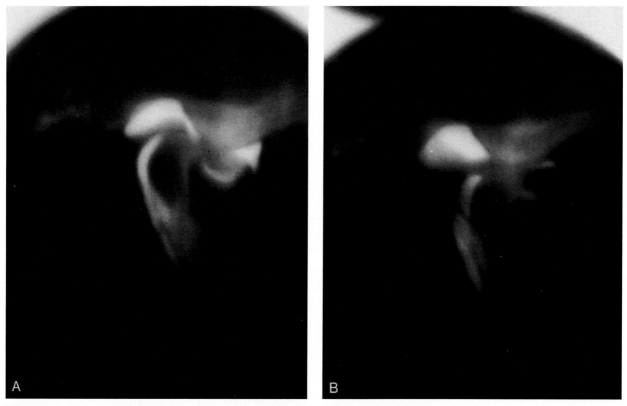

FIGURE 7–4 / Arthrotomographs showing the anterior position of the disk when the jaw was in a closed relationship (*A*) and an open relationship (*B*). (Note the clear failure of the disk to rotate posteriorly as the condyle translates.)

Analysis of Jaw Movement

The jaw movement variables in this study were maximum active (unassisted) opening, maximum passive (assisted) opening, and maximum right and left lateral movement. The opening movement was assessed with a metric ruler (mm) placed interincisally at the right central incisors (Fig. 7–5). Incisal overbite, measured in a position of maximum intercuspation, was then added to the interincisal measurement. A mark corresponding to the mandibular incisor midline was made on the maxillary incisors, and the ruler was again used to assess the maximum amount of active lateral movement produced by each patient.

A jaw-tracking system was also used at each examination on every patient to assess the overall envelope of motion in the frontal plane (Fig. 7–6). A light-emitting diode (LED) was fixed to the mandibular incisors, and a camera sensor was attached to a special helmet apparatus so that neither the source nor the sensor impeded mandibular movement or function in any way. The camera was positioned 120 mm away and directly in front of the LED, which was always attached so that it was parallel to the occlusal plane and in line with the mandibular midline. This system is accurate to 5 percent and is linear up to 50 mm of movement. To track the frontal envelope of motion, the patient was instructed to move fully to the right, then to stay fully to the right and open as wide as possible, then to close and move fully to the left, then to stay fully to the left and open as wide as possible, and then to close. These movements were performed twice at each visit, and the movement recorded was then plotted and the area determined by x-y digitization.

Analysis of Joint Sounds

Patients were questioned regarding their history and the current status of any temporomandibular joint sounds. The presence or absence of joint sounds was evaluated by light digital palpation during jaw movement and sounds were noted to be absent, slight (barely noticeable), or present. If multiple sounds or crepitation sounds were present in any single movement, they were noted in the same manner.

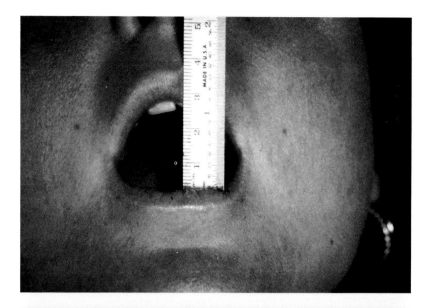

FIGURE 7–5 / A ruler is used to measure interincisal distance during maximum active opening.

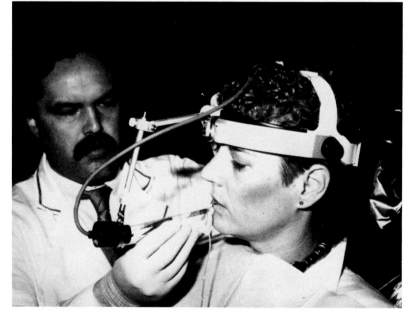

FIGURE 7–6 / A jaw-tracking device in place on a patient. The light sensor is being positioned at the correct distance from the light to record movement in the frontal plane.

Assessment of Pain

Patients assessed their pain by using a standard 100-mm visual analog scale (Fig. 7–7), along which a mark was placed to indicate the amount of usual pain during the previous week. An eight-item jaw pain questionnaire was also used; this allowed the patient to rate the pain in different areas of the jaw and at different times of the day (Fig. 7–8, Part A).

Assessment of Jaw Function

Each time the patient was assessed during the study, function was rated by using both a 5-item jaw function questionnaire and a general 18-item questionnaire regarding any limitation of daily activities (Fig. 7–8, Part B, and Fig. 7–9). The 5-item questionnaire asked about frequency of joint noises, locking, and difficulty in opening. The 18-item daily activity questionnaire asked about pain that occurred with various activities of daily living.

Rate the INTENSITY of your USUAL PAIN during the LAST WEEK by placing a slash (/) somewhere on the line below.

No pain   Most intense
pain imaginable

FIGURE 7–7 / A 100-mm visual analog scale used to assess pain.

JAW SYMPTOM QUESTIONNAIRE

Name: _____   Date: _____

INSTRUCTIONS: Please check the appropriate answer to the following questions.

A. Jaw Pain Questions	Doesn't Hurt At All	Hurts A Little	Hurts A Lot	Almost Unbearable	Unbearable Pain Without Relief
1. Does it hurt when you open wide or yawn?	_____	_____	_____	_____	_____
2. Does it hurt when you chew, or use the jaws?	_____	_____	_____	_____	_____
3. Does it hurt when you are not chewing or using the jaws?	_____	_____	_____	_____	_____
4. Is your pain worse on waking?	_____	_____	_____	_____	_____
5. Do you have pain in front of the ears or ear aches?	_____	_____	_____	_____	_____
6. Do you have jaw muscle (cheek) pain?	_____	_____	_____	_____	_____
7. Do you have pain in the temples?	_____	_____	_____	_____	_____
8. Do you have pain or soreness in the teeth?	_____	_____	_____	_____	_____

B. Jaw Function Questions	No	Maybe A Little	Quite A Lot	Almost All The Time	All the Time Without Stopping
1. Do your jaw joints make noise so that it bothers you or others?	_____	_____	_____	_____	_____
2. Do you find it difficult to open your mouth wide?	_____	_____	_____	_____	_____
3. Does your jaw ever get stuck (lock) as you open it?	_____	_____	_____	_____	_____
4. Does your jaw ever lock open so you cannot close it?	_____	_____	_____	_____	_____
5. Is your bite uncomfortable?	_____	_____	_____	_____	_____

FIGURE 7–8 / Part A of this questionnaire is used to assess pain level in the jaw, and part B is used to assess the ability of the jaw to function.

ACTIVITY LIMITATION SCALE

Name: _____   Date: _____

INSTRUCTIONS: Please check in the columns below how much these activities USUALLY CAUSE PAIN (does not include unusual or prolonged activity, e.g., driving on a long trip).

Activity	Doesn't Hurt At All	Hurts A Little	Hurts A Lot	Almost Unbearable	Unbearable Pain Prevents Activity
1. Walking	_____	_____	_____	_____	_____
2. Eating Soft Food	_____	_____	_____	_____	_____
3. Eating Hard Food	_____	_____	_____	_____	_____
4. Jaw Opening	_____	_____	_____	_____	_____
5. Sleeping	_____	_____	_____	_____	_____
6. Chewing	_____	_____	_____	_____	_____
7. Swallowing	_____	_____	_____	_____	_____
8. Talking	_____	_____	_____	_____	_____
9. Pushing & Pulling	_____	_____	_____	_____	_____
10. Resting	_____	_____	_____	_____	_____
11. Driving	_____	_____	_____	_____	_____
12. Dressing	_____	_____	_____	_____	_____
13. Sports	_____	_____	_____	_____	_____
14. Reading	_____	_____	_____	_____	_____
15. Watching TV	_____	_____	_____	_____	_____
16. Household Chores	_____	_____	_____	_____	_____
17. Gardening	_____	_____	_____	_____	_____
18. Employment	_____	_____	_____	_____	_____

FIGURE 7–9 / This 18-item questionnaire was used to assess the effect the patient's jaw pain and dysfunction had on daily activities.

Prior Treatment

Each patient was also individually interviewed, and from these sessions, the following presurgical treatment characteristics emerged. Before seeing the surgeon for arthroscopic treatment, each of these subjects had been treated for their TMJ problem by an average of 2.1 doctors. The patients had been in treatment for an average of 11.5 months before this surgery, and they had had their TMJ problem for an average of 43.8 months. Four of the six patients had been in a state of closed locking for less than 10 months before the preoperative appointment, and the other two reported several episodes of prior locking and a current locking episode that had lasted for more than one year.

Radiographic Observations

One of the six patients studied exhibited radiographic evidence of moderate TMJ osteoarthrosis, which resulted in condylar flattening and a mildly decreased joint space. Another of these patients exhibited a clear and noticeable bony spur on the anterior slope of the condyle. The other four patients had no significant osseous abnormalities, flattening, or bony spurs. All arthrographic reports revealed that disk displacement without reduction existed to some degree in each case reported here. Four showed partial condyle-disk translation, whereas two showed clearly reduced superior joint space filling and no disk movement with condyle translation.

Results of Treatment for Closed Lock
Jaw Movement

Maximum active opening ability increased, on the average, 15 mm, from 26.3 mm to 41.5 mm (Fig. 7–10). The maximum passive opening ability exhibited a mean change of 14 mm, increasing from 29.8 mm to 43.0 mm. Lateral movement ability, which was 7.3 mm on the right and 7.8 mm on the left preoperatively, increased slightly (1.5 mm on the right and 1.7 mm on the left). In that the lateral movement was not severely limited before surgery, this amount of increase in lateral movement is not remarkable. The total area of the frontal envelope of motion increased an average of 62 percent for these patients (Fig. 7–11A and B).

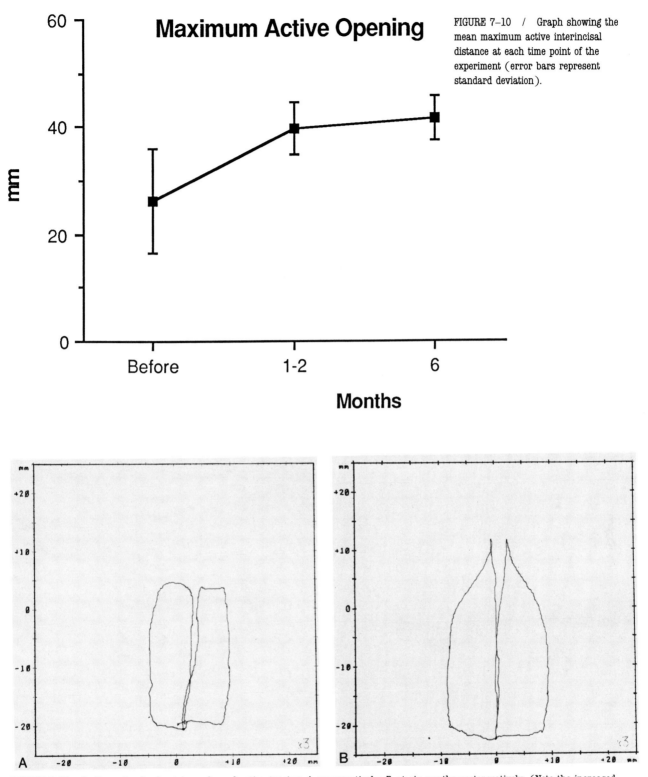

FIGURE 7–10 / Graph showing the mean maximum active interincisal distance at each time point of the experiment (error bars represent standard deviation).

FIGURE 7–11 / Example of a frontal envelope-of-motion tracing: *A*, preoperatively; *B*, at six months postoperatively. (Note the increased range of motion postoperatively.)

Jaw Pain

On the 100-mm scale, the patients rated the intensity of their usual preoperative pain at an average value of 48.5 mm; six months postoperatively it was rated at 11.8 mm, a decrease of 36.7 mm (i.e., a 75.7 percent decrease) in usual pain intensity (Fig. 7–12). Average total scores on the jaw pain questionnaire (with possible scoring from 0 to 32) decreased from 13.8 to 5.0 (an average decrease of 63.8 percent) (Fig. 7–13).

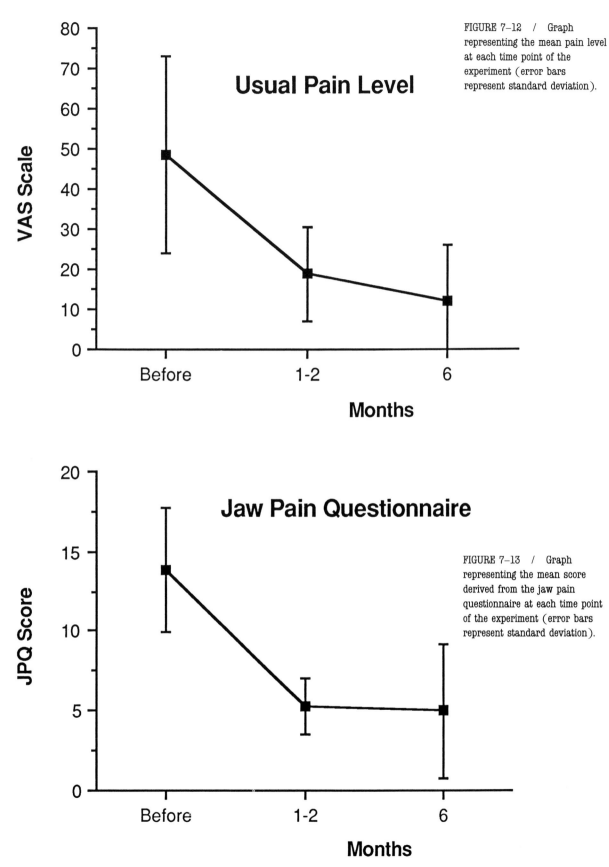

FIGURE 7–12 / Graph representing the mean pain level at each time point of the experiment (error bars represent standard deviation).

FIGURE 7–13 / Graph representing the mean score derived from the jaw pain questionnaire at each time point of the experiment (error bars represent standard deviation).

Jaw Function

The daily activity limitation scale, with a possible score of 0 to 72, showed a decrease from 17.8 to 4.8 (a 73.0 percent decrease) on the average, and patient responses on the jaw function questionnaire, with a possible score of 0 to 20, showed an average decrease from 9.2 (preoperatively) to 2.6 (postoperatively), a 71.7 percent average decrease (Figs. 7–14 and 7–15).

Joint Sounds

Before treatment, none of the patients exhibited clicking and only one patient had evidence of crepitation in the locked joint. Six months after treatment, definite TMJ clicking noises were present in one patient, slight joint clicking noises were present in three patients, and mild crepitation at the six-month postoperative examination was present in another patient. Only one patient had no joint sounds at the six-month examination, and the patient with crepitation preoperatively still had crepitation postoperatively.

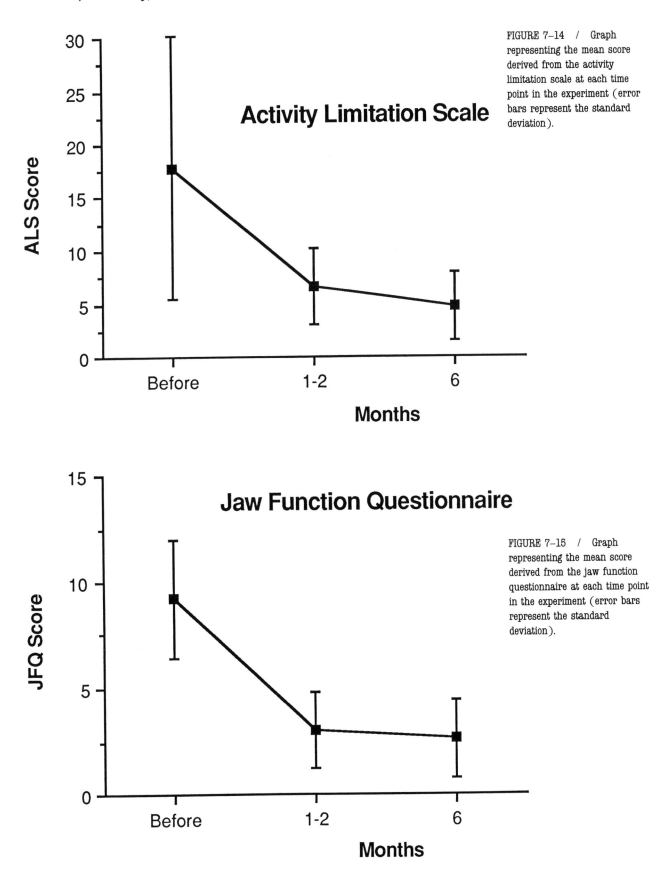

FIGURE 7–14 / Graph representing the mean score derived from the activity limitation scale at each time point in the experiment (error bars represent the standard deviation).

FIGURE 7–15 / Graph representing the mean score derived from the jaw function questionnaire at each time point in the experiment (error bars represent the standard deviation).

Overall Assessment of Treatment

The results for these patients showed an impressive increase in mobility, decrease in pain, and increase in functional ability by six months postoperatively. The results perhaps would have been even better had only patients with acute or subacute closed lock (of less than 10 months' duration) without any significant osteoarthrotic changes been treated.

Patients were told that it was not a goal of the procedure to stop joint sounds, and although noises were present postoperatively, they were apparently not of much concern to the patients and did not seem to be interfering with postoperative function.

Patients were generally quite pleased with their treatment. Only one of the six still exhibited reduced mobility (opening less than 38 mm), and one other still reported pain greater than 20 on the 100-mm visual analog scale. This patient was the one who exhibited crepitation preoperatively and noticeable flattening of the condyle on the tomograms.

This preliminary report includes only 6 completed cases out of 16 currently being studied. The overall results for these six cases were surprisingly good, however. The value of arthroscopic surgery for acute and subacute closed locking relative to other treatment methods has not yet been established. These data, however, have encouraged further research. The remarkable success of this procedure and the relatively slight invasiveness of the technique suggest that the mechanism of reduced condyle translation may be more a result of disk adherence than of disk displacement. If so, then the need for surgical repositioning of the disk is a concept in need of re-evaluation. Preliminary findings in the study described suggest that it is not necessary to reposition the disk physically (i.e., surgically) to re-establish translation.

In summary, arthroscopic surgery for acute and (to a lesser extent) chronic closed locking produced a dramatic decrease in pain, an increase in mobility, and an improvement in function. Residual symptoms of reduced mobility and pain were associated with preoperative osteoarthrotic changes. If TMJ clicking and crepitation sounds were present before surgery, they were also present postoperatively, and no significant morbidity was encountered as a result of this procedure.

Acknowledgment

All pre- and postoperative measurements of the six subjects participating in an ongoing study of arthroscopic surgical treatment were made at the UCLA Dental Research Institute's Clinical Research Center. Preoperative radiographs were evaluated by a member of the UCLA Oral Radiology Department.

References

Alpern MC, Nuelle DG, Ufema JW: Direct parasagittal computed tomography and arthroscopic surgery of the temporomandibular joint. Angle Orthod 56:91–101, 1986.

Burke RH: Temporomandibular joint diagnosis: Arthroscopy. J Craniomandib Pract 3:233–235, 1985.

Donlon WC: TMJ arthroscopy: Problem or panacea (letter). J Oral Maxillofac Surg 45:2, 1987.

Hellsing G, Holmlund A, Nordenram A, Wredmark T: Arthroscopy of the temporomandibular joint. Examination of 2 patients with suspected disk derangement. Int J Oral Surg 13:69–74, 1984.

Hellsing G, Lestrange P, Holmlund A: Temporomandibular-mandibular joint disorders: A diagnostic challenge. J Prosthet Dent 56:600–606, 1986.

Hilsabeck RB, Laskin DM: Arthroscopy of the temporomandibular joint of the rabbit. J Oral Surg 36:938–943, 1978.

Holmlund A, Hellsing G: Arthroscopy of the temporomandibular joint. An autopsy study. Int J Oral Surg 14:169–175, 1985.

Holmlund A, Hellsing G, Wredmark T: Arthroscopy of the temporomandibular joint. A clinical study. Int J Oral Maxillofac Surg 15:715–721, 1986.

Kino K: Morphological and structural observation of the synovial membranes and their folds relating to the endoscopic findings in the upper cavity of the human temporomandibular joint. J Stomatol Soc Jpn 47:98, 1980.

Kino K, Ohnishi M, Shioda S, Ichijo T: Morphological observation on the inner surface of the temporomandibular joint: Histological investigation relating to the arthroscopic findings in the upper cavity. Jpn J Oral Surg 27:1379, 1981.

Laskin D: Arthroscope effective for diagnosing TMJ diseases (interview). Ill Dent J 50:259, 1981.

Murakami K, Hoshino K: Regional anatomical nomenclature and arthroscopic terminology in human temporomandibular joints. Okajimas Folia Anat Jpn 58:745–760, 1982.

Murakami K, Ito K: Arthroscopy of the temporomandibular joint: Arthroscopic anatomy and arthroscopic approaches in the human cadaver. Arthroscopy 6:1–13, 1981 (in Japanese, abstract in English).

Murakami K, Ito K: Arthroscopy of the temporomandibular joint, in Watanabe M (ed): Arthroscopy of Small Joints. Tokyo, Igaku Shoin, 1985.

Murakami KI, Iizuka T, Matsuki M, Ono T: Diagnostic arthroscopy of the TMJ: Differential diagnoses in patients with limited jaw opening. J Craniomandib Pract 4:117–126, 1986.

Murakami K, Matsuki M, Iizuka T, Ono T, Hoshino T: Arthroscopic differential diagnoses and treatments of the locking symptoms of the temporomandibular joint and their regional anatomical interpretations. Proceedings of the 7th Congress of European Association for Maxillofacial Surgery, Paris, 1984, Abstr 89.

Murakami K, Matsumoto K, Iizuka T: Suppurative arthritis of the temporomandibular joint. Report of a case with special reference to arthroscopic observations. J Maxillofac Surg 12:41–45, 1984.

Murakami K, Ono T: Temporomandibular joint arthroscopy by inferolateral approach. Int J Oral Maxillofac Surg 15:401–407, 1986.

Nuelle DG, Alpern MC: Arthroscopic debridement of an arthritic TMJ. Fla Dent J 57:4–5, 44, 1986.

Ohnishi M: Arthroscopy of the temporomandibular joint. J Stomatol Soc Jpn 42: 207–213, 1975.

Ohnishi M: Clinical application of arthroscopy in the temporomandibular joint diseases. Bull Tokyo Med Dent Univ 27:141–150, 1980.

Sanders B: Arthroscopic surgery of the temporomandibular joint: Treatment of internal derangement with persistent closed lock. Oral Surg Oral Med Oral Pathol 62:361–372, 1986.

Sanders B, Buoncristiani R. Diagnostic and surgical arthroscopy of the temporomandibular joint: Clinical experience with 137 procedures over a 2-year period. J. Craniomandib Disord 1:202–213, 1987.

Ufema JW: TMJ arthroscopic update. Another look at CT scans. Fla Dent J 57: 15, 47, 1986.

Ufema JW, Alpern MC, Nuelle DG: Corrected parasagittal direct CT imaging of the temporomandibular joint. With arthroscopic correlation. Angle Orthod 56:102–117, 1986.

Williams RA, Laskin DM: Arthroscopic examination of experimentally induced pathologic conditions of the rabbit temporomandibular joint. J Oral Surg 38:652–659, 1980.

8 Treatment Planning /

John B. Ross
Bruce Sanders
Ken-Ichiro Murakami

The full possibilities for examination and treatment of the temporomandibular joint with arthroscopy are still being explored, and a combination of arthroscopic procedures with other methods of treatment is a necessary part of this development. Diagnostic categories for common temporomandibular joint disorders have been delineated in conjunction with plans for arthroscopic examination and for treatment that includes not only arthroscopic procedures but also other treatment modalities.

The treatment plans discussed here are only hypothetical. They have been developed in accordance with the surgical techniques and diagnostic procedures described in Chapters 4, 5, and 6.

The first three categories of disorders that have been studied are anteriorly displaced disk with reduction (Fig. 8–1), anteriorly displaced disk without reduction (Fig. 8–2), and osteoarthrosis and arthritis (Fig. 8–3). All have the common feature of significant pain and dysfunction, and all of the arthroscopic treatment plans have been proposed subsequent to failure of initial treatment modalities and after an appropriate radiographic examination has taken place.

ANTERIORLY DISPLACED DISK (ADD) WITH
REDUCTION (PAINFUL CLICKING JOINT)

Significant pain and dysfunction

Negative results on screening film

Patient refractory to nonsurgical treatment

Arthrogram to confirm diagonsis of ADD with reduction and to assess
morphology and associated pathology

Arthroscopic examination to confirm diagnosis and assess morphology
and associated pathology (such as surface adhesions)

(or)

Arthroscopic lysis and lavage   Arthrotomy with disk repair
Disk and mandibular manipulation

Return to nonsurgical treatment

FIGURE 8–1   /   Treatment plan for the patient with anteriorly displaced disk with reduction.

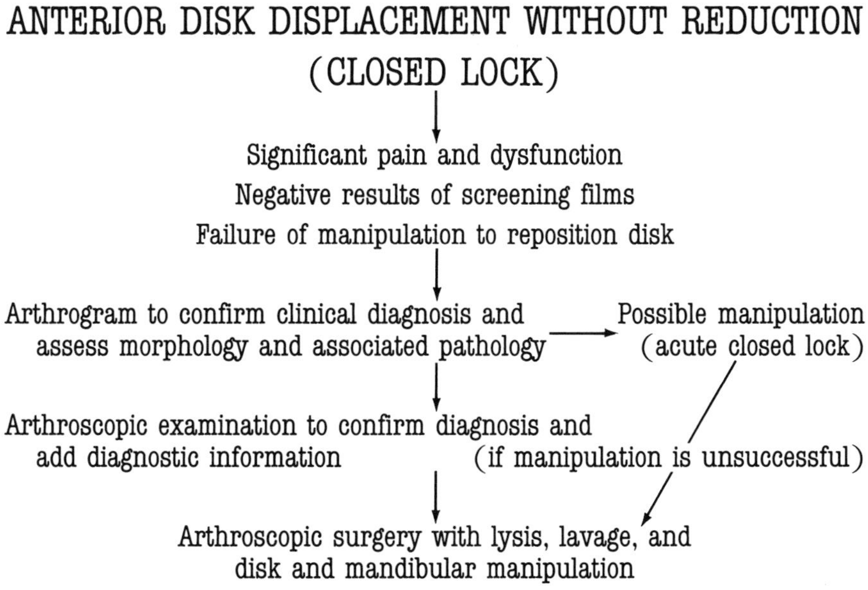

ANTERIOR DISK DISPLACEMENT WITHOUT REDUCTION
(CLOSED LOCK)

Significant pain and dysfunction
Negative results of screening films
Failure of manipulation to reposition disk

Arthrogram to confirm clinical diagnosis and   Possible manipulation
assess morphology and associated pathology   (acute closed lock)

Arthroscopic examination to confirm diagnosis and
add diagnostic information   (if manipulation is unsuccessful)

Arthroscopic surgery with lysis, lavage, and
disk and mandibular manipulation

FIGURE 8–2 / Treatment plan for the patient with anteriorly displaced disk without reduction.

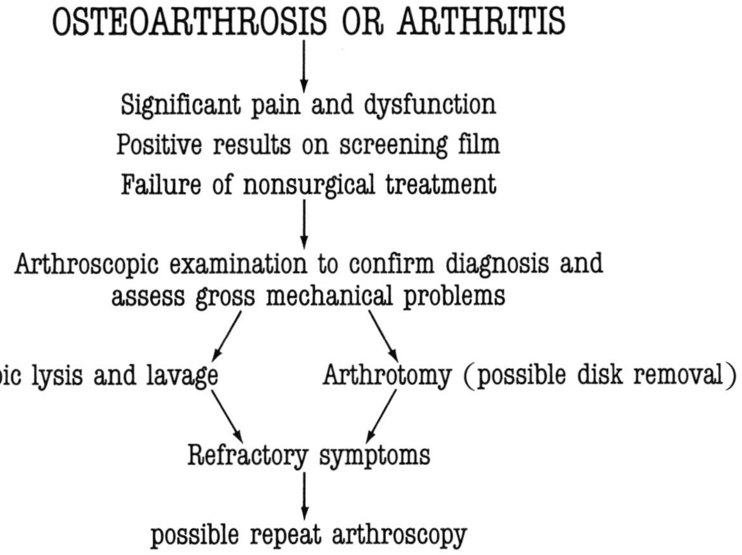

OSTEOARTHROSIS OR ARTHRITIS

Significant pain and dysfunction
Positive results on screening film
Failure of nonsurgical treatment

Arthroscopic examination to confirm diagnosis and
assess gross mechanical problems

Arthroscopic lysis and lavage   Arthrotomy (possible disk removal)

Refractory symptoms

possible repeat arthroscopy

FIGURE 8–3 / Treatment plan for the patient with osteoarthritis or arthritis.

Appropriate radiographic examination begins with a temporomandibular joint series. In the case of a disk displacement, no significant bony abnormalities would be expected, but in the case of osteoarthrosis or arthritis involving the joint, characteristic radiographic signs would be seen. The soft tissue disorders of disk displacement would be further evaluated with arthrography to confirm the clinical diagnosis, to assess morphological aspects of the soft tissue, and to delineate the associated disorders completely.

The radiographic examinations would be followed by the arthroscopic examination to confirm and add diagnostic information, particularly about surface adhesions or other types of surface disorders. It would also help to assess gross mechanical problems. At this point the surgeon would make a final decision as to whether to proceed with arthroscopic surgery and its associated lavage or to choose an open surgical procedure of the appropriate type. Should the arthroscopic surgery provide no long-term relief of symptoms, then the possibility of open surgical repair is still available. With arthroscopic success, the patient would be returned to nonsurgical modalities of therapy.

During the arthroscopic examination of a temporomandibular joint with an anteriorly displaced disk without reduction, if it is determined that arthroscopy alone cannot fully mobilize the joint, the patient would immediately undergo the appropriate open surgical procedure. Failure to reposition the disk is not, however, an indication to proceed to open surgery. The type of open surgery of the soft tissue components, whether a disk repair or a disk removal, would be determined in part by their morphological and pathological features.

One of the great advantages of the arthroscopic surgical procedure is that it is significantly less traumatic to both the joint and the patient than an open procedure. Should an arthroscopic surgical correction be done with only limited success, the option to do an open surgical treatment at a future date is available.

Two other categories of temporomandibular joint disorders that are appropriate for arthroscopic examination and surgery involve the postarthrotomy patient with temporomandibular joint pain and dysfunction (Fig. 8–4) and the patient with temporomandibular joint pain that has been refractory to other diagnostic modalities (Fig. 8–5). In the case of a patient who presents after arthrotomy with a significantly decreased range of motion and pain, the arthroscope can be valuable both as an examination and as a treatment tool. In cases in which soft tissue repair was the surgical treatment, an arthrogram would first be done to assess the current joint form and function. The arthrographic findings could lead in some cases, such as adhesions, to an arthroscopic lysis and lavage procedure. In other cases, they should rule out significant intercapsular joint disorders and indicate a return to nonsurgical treatment.

POST-ARTHROTOMY (PAIN AND DECREASED RANGE OF MOTION)
DISK REPAIR
(or disk removed without implant)
Arthroscopic examination
Arthroscopic lysis and lavage
Return to nonsurgical treatment
DISK REMOVAL WITH IMPLANT
Partial arthrotomy to remove implant
Arthroscopic examination
of pseudo disk fibrous barrier)
Arthroscopic lysis and lavage
Reconstructive surgery

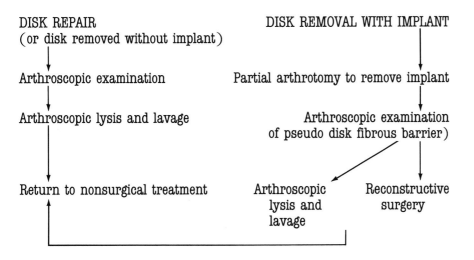

FIGURE 8–4 / Treatment plan for the patient with postarthrotomy temporomandibular joint pain and decreased range of motion.

TMJ PAIN REFRACTORY TO TREATMENT
Inconclusive examination results
Negative results on screening film
Decreased symptoms after lidocaine wash of TMJ
Trial nonsurgical treatment
Arthrogram
Diagnosis and treatment
Perforation or
no significant findings
Arthroscopic examination
Positive results
Negative results
No surgical treatment
Perforations (assess size, site,
and associated pathology)
Adhesive capsulitis
Morphological changes
Arthroscopic lysis and lavage
(or possible arthrotomy)

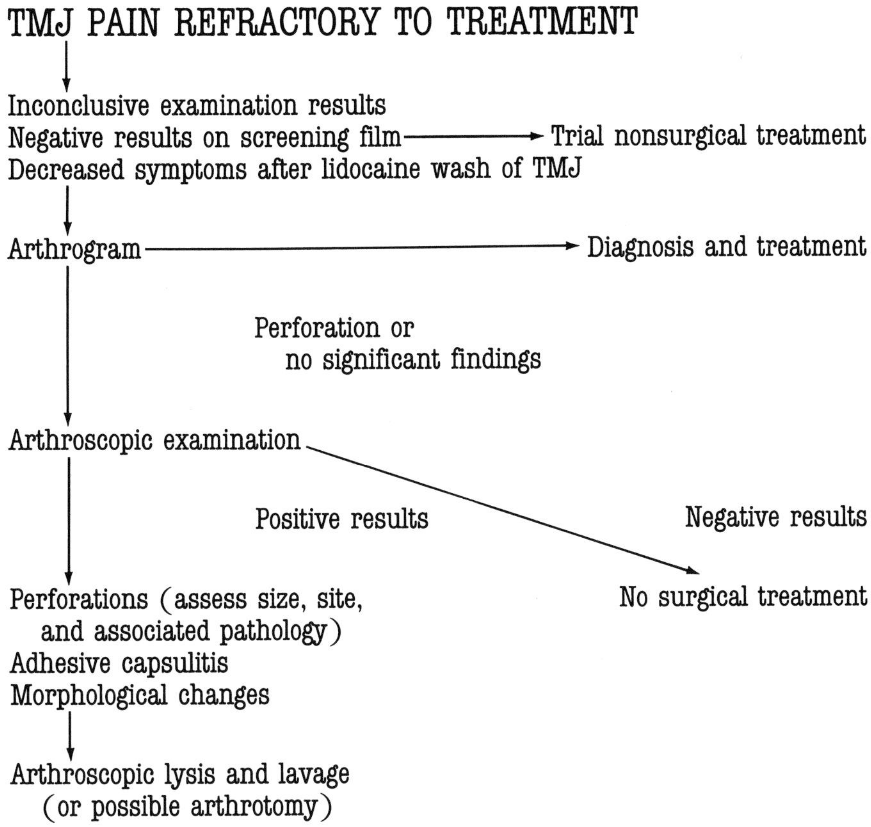

FIGURE 8–5 / Treatment plan for the patient with temporomandibular joint pain refractory to treatment.

In cases in which an implant has been placed in the joint or the arthrographic results indicate a need for either arthroscopic examination or surgery, the arthroscopic examination would be the next step. The arthroscope is unique in its ability to assess the position of the implant and associated incapsulation. It is also useful in assessing any associated disorder in such a joint. Following the arthroscopic examination, the surgeon would have the option of continuing with either arthroscopic or open surgery.

Intercapsular temporomandibular joint pain that has been refractory to other modalities of diagnosis and treatment may be considered for diagnostic arthroscopy. If the results of arthroscopic examination are positive for a specific pathological entity (i.e., synovitis, adhesion, and so forth), then appropriate treatment can be rendered. The arthroscopic examination is useful in evaluating perforations, particularly in terms of the site, size, and pathological change associated with such lesions.

In cases of intercapsular pain that cannot be diagnosed because of inconclusive examination findings and negative results on a screening film, a lidocaine wash of the joint may be appropriate. If the anesthetic reduces or eliminates the intercapsular symptoms, a trial of nonsurgical therapy is indicated. Should this therapy not add any new information, an arthrogram should be performed. If the arthrogram reveals no significant findings or if a perforation is noted, then the patient should proceed to the arthroscopic examination.

The clinical use of the arthroscope in the examination and treatment of temporomandibular joint disorders is rapidly evolving, and the flow charts presented here were generated in the infancy of the technique. As the procedure evolves along with its technical possibilities, the clinical use of the procedure will also evolve and its place and role in the patient's overall treatment plan will continue to change.

9 Comparative Imaging Study / Carol A. Bibb
Andrew G. Pullinger
Fernando Baldioceda
Ken-Ichiro Murakami
John B. Ross

As new TMJ imaging technologies become available, the clinician is faced with increasingly complex decisions in the selection of diagnostic procedures. Comparison of the strengths and limitations of various procedures under experimental conditions must be made to establish appropriate selection criteria. Two of these procedures, tomography and arthrotomography, are established examinations, whereas arthroscopy has only recently been applied to the temporomandibular joint. This problem of selection has been recently studied by independent experienced clinicians who also evaluated the resulting diagnostic data. Their findings were compared among the three imaging techniques and subsequently to the findings at anatomical dissection.

To compare these imaging techniques, six hemisected embalmed cadaver heads (stored frozen when not being studied) were examined in the following order:

Tomography. Axially corrected tomography was carried out with a Phillips Polytome to obtain lateral, central, and medial third sections of the joints. Because orientation of the hemisected material in the craniostat was less than ideal, a scout film was used to provide the most axially correct image.

Arthrotomography. Prior to imaging, the material was softened overnight in a 10 percent formalin solution to improve condylar movement. Upper and lower joint spaces were injected with contrast medium, and the filling of each space was observed under fluoroscopy. Arthrograms in the tomographic mode were prepared in both open and closed positions to the extent that mobility of the cadaver material permitted.

Arthroscopy. Diagnostic arthroscopy was next performed by using a Watanabe No. 24 arthroscope (Olympus Selfoscope) with a diameter of 1.7 mm. The inferolateral approach was used to examine the upper joint compartment. In addition, inspection of the lower joint space was attempted in all cases.

Dissection. At the completion of the arthroscopic examination, the joints were dissected. Sagittal cuts were made through the lateral and medial poles of the condyle, leaving a central block approximately 1 cm thick.

An independent report was prepared for each procedure by the examiner, who had no knowledge of the other findings. Each examiner also rated each joint as normal or abnormal on the basis of his or her examination.

Findings of the Joint Analysis

Tables 9–1 through 9–3 summarize findings in the six joints categorized under osseous changes, disk displacement, and disk perforation. Table 9–4 shows the normalcy rating for each joint, as determined by the examiner performing each technique. The scores varied with technique, except for Joint 2, which displayed the most extreme changes (Fig. 9–1).

TABLE 9–1

Osseous Changes

JOINT	TOMOGRAPHY	ARTHROGRAPHY	ARTHROSCOPY	DISSECTION
1				X
2	X		X	X
3				X
4	X			X
5	X			X
6	X			X

TABLE 9-2
Disk Displacement

JOINT	ARTHROGRAPHY	ARTHROSCOPY	DISSECTION
1	X	X	X
2	X	X	X
3	?	X	X
4	X		X
5	X	X	X
6		X	X

?Could not be diagnosed due to joint immobility.

TABLE 9-3
Disk Perforation

JOINT	ARTHROGRAPHY	ARTHROSCOPY	DISSECTION
1			
2	X	X	X
3	X	X	X
4			
5			X
6			

TABLE 9-4
Normal/Abnormal Ratings

JOINT	TOMOGRAPHY	ARTHROGRAPHY	ARTHROSCOPY	DISSECTION
1	0	2	3	2
2	3	3	3	3
3	0	1	3	1
4	3	3	0	1
5	1	3	2	2
6	1	0	2	2

0   1 2 3
Normal. . . . . Abnormal

Tomography was considered the technique of choice for diagnosing osseous changes in the condyle and temporal component (Table 9–1). All six joints showed such changes at dissection. Tomography allowed diagnosis of osseous changes in four of these joints (Fig. 9–2), whereas arthroscopy revealed only the very gross osseous changes seen in Joint 2.

Arthrotomography was found to be useful for diagnosing disk displacement (Table 9–2). All six joints had some degree of disk displacement at dissection. Four were diagnosed by arthrography (Fig. 9–3), one could not be diagnosed because of joint immobility, and one was incorrectly diagnosed as normal. When both joint spaces were injected, this technique was also able to reveal articular disk morphology as it appeared in the sagittal plane. It was difficult to examine bony contours using arthrotomography, however, because of the filling of the lateral aspects of the joint spaces with contrast. In addition, this technique allowed correct diagnosis of perforations (Fig. 9–3) in two of the three joints that showed perforations at dissection (Table 9–3).

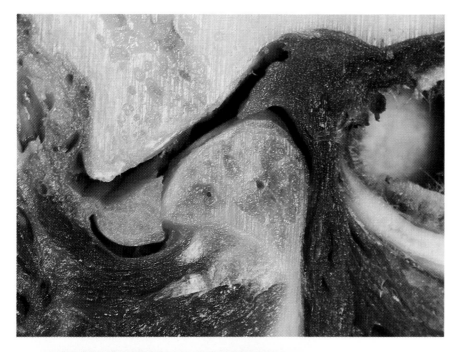

FIGURE 9–1 / Sagittal section through the central part of Joint 2 at dissection. Note the extensive osseous changes on the condyle and articular eminence. There is an anteriorly displaced disk and a large perforation.

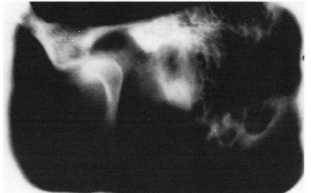

FIGURE 9–2 / Sagittal tomogram through the central part of Joint 2. Note the proliferative remodeling on the anterior aspect of the condyle, the very thin condylar neck, and the flattening of the articular eminence.

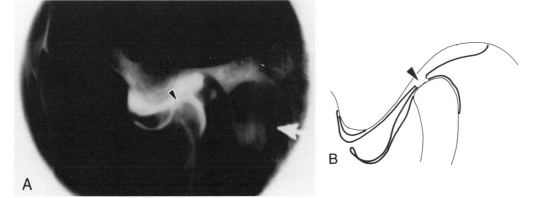

FIGURE 9–3 / Sagittal arthrotomogram (A) and diagram (B) through the central part of Joint 2, revealing an anteriorly displaced disk and a large perforation (arrow). Note that the filling of the joint spaces with contrast dye obscures the bony contours visualized in the tomogram (Fig. 9–2).

Arthroscopy provided a narrow, continuous image of surface morphology (Fig. 9–4). Disk displacement was correctly diagnosed in five out of the six joints (Table 9–2). Disk displacement was inferred, however, from associated disorders such as stretching of the posterior attachment (Fig. 9–5) rather than by direct observation. Perforations were correctly diagnosed in two of the three joints that showed perforations at dissection (Table 9–3). Arthroscopy provided the most information about the location and size of perforations and associated pathological change (Fig. 9–6).

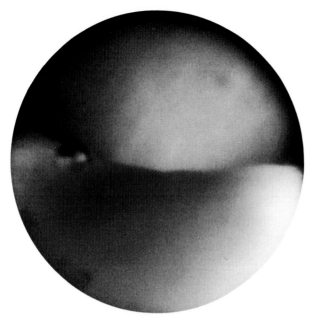

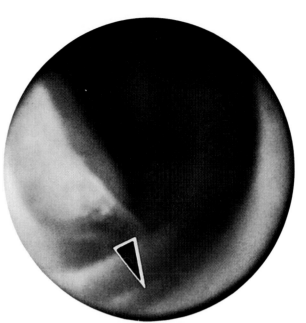

FIGURE 9–4 / Normal arthroscopic view of the upper joint compartment of Joint 4, showing the smooth articular surfaces of the articular eminence (*above*) and the disk (*below*). Anterior is to the right.

FIGURE 9–5 / Arthroscopic view of the upper joint compartment of Joint 3. Note the stretched posterior attachment (*arrow*). This suggests anterior disk displacement, although the actual position and morphology of the disk are not visualized.

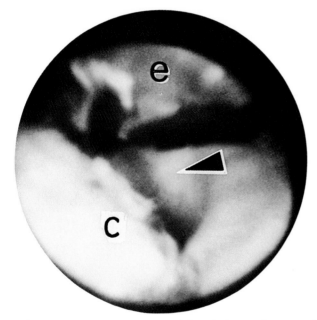

FIGURE 9–6 / Arthroscopic view of Joint 2, showing the ruptured anterior end of the disk (*arrow*). Note the irregularity of the articular surface of both the anterior aspect of the condyle (c) and the articular eminence (e).

Certain anatomical features were apparent only in joint *dissection* where inspection was direct, thorough, and multidimensional. Both osseous and soft tissues together with their relationships were visualized. For example, there was a proliferation of soft tissue on the posterior-superior aspect of the condyle of Joint 1 (Fig. 9–7), which otherwise went undetected. In the dissected joint the dramatic differences in disk morphology and position from lateral to medial were revealed (Fig. 9–8). Furthermore, it was possible to examine the extreme lateral aspect of the joint. The lateral disk perforation in Joint 5, which was not revealed by arthrography or arthroscopy, was found on dissection.

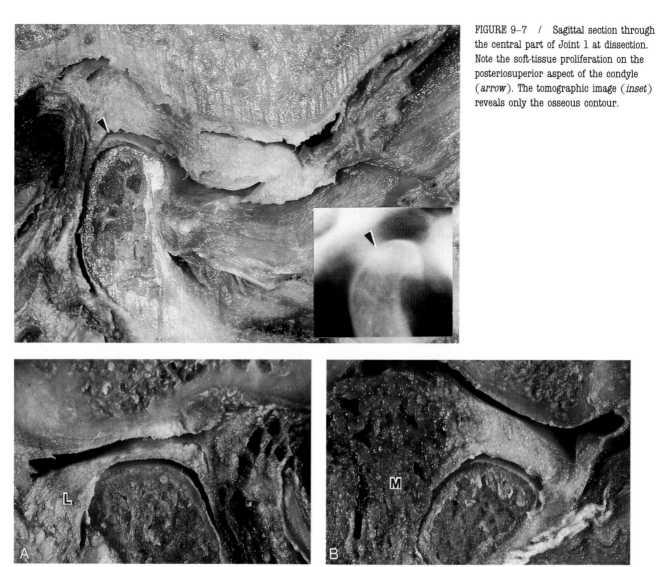

FIGURE 9–7 / Sagittal section through the central part of Joint 1 at dissection. Note the soft-tissue proliferation on the posteriosuperior aspect of the condyle (*arrow*). The tomographic image (*inset*) reveals only the osseous contour.

FIGURE 9–8 / Sagittal sections through the lateral (L) and medial (M) parts of Joint 3. Note the variability in the position and thickness of the disk.

Interpreting the Value of Imaging Techniques

The results of this preliminary investigation underscore the importance of selecting a TMJ imaging technique on the basis of clinical findings. Although each technique has value, none is comprehensive. Furthermore, some anatomical features cannot be revealed by any of the currently available techniques. This comparative study provided information on features best diagnosed by each technique and the limitations of each.

The extensive degree of morphologic change in this sample facilitates comparisons between the imaging techniques and underscores the low incidence of false-negative diagnoses (Tables 9–1 through 9–3). On the other hand, it was impossible to determine the incidence of false-positive diagnoses for osseous changes or disk displacement because all six joints showed such changes at dissection (Tables 9–1 and 9–2). There were no false-positive results for disk perforation as diagnosed by arthrography or arthroscopy (Table 9–3). Information on false-positive findings is especially important in any diagnostic technique that could lead to a decision for surgery.

Examination of the false-negative diagnoses provides insight into the diagnostic limitations of these techniques. The lateral aspect of the joint is particularly difficult to observe through imaging. The two joints with osseous changes undetected by tomography had relatively minimal osseous changes localized to the lateral portions of the condyle and temporal bone. Eckerdal (1973) has reported that the tomographic representation of actual morphology is most distorted laterally and medially, especially for the condyle. Similarly, the disk perforation that went undiagnosed by arthrography and arthroscopy was located in the lateral aspect. This agrees with the findings of Liedberg and Westesson (1986), in which perforations not diagnosed by arthroscopy were usually in the lateral part of the joint. It is unfortunate that the morphology of the lateral portion of the joint cannot be more accurately imaged in that the lateral third has been reported to have the highest incidence of disk thinning (Hansson et al., 1977), osteoarthrosis (Westesson and Rohlin, 1984), and deviation in form (Solberg et al., 1985).

Currently, no clinical imaging technique adequately reveals the articular soft tissue that covers the osseous components of the condyle and temporal bone. It is clear that the outlines of the bone and soft tissue are not predictably congruent (Baldioceda et al., 1987; Pullinger et al., 1987). Therefore, the conventional tomographic image of the condyle and temporal component does not portray the actual articular surfaces well even in the face of significant osseous defects. Conversely, arthroscopy reveals surface morphology (in the upper compartment) but does not show the relationship of the soft tissue to the underlying bone.

Arthrography has been the accepted standard imaging technique for the diagnosis of disk displacement (Helms et al., 1984; Ross, 1987). In this study, there were two false-negative findings of disk displacement, one of which was largely a technique problem due to overall joint immobility. The application of computed tomography (CT) and magnetic resonance imaging (MRI) to diagnose disk displacement has advantages, but at this time it may carry a high false-positive rate: 4 percent for CT (Helms et al., 1984) and 23 percent for MRI (Katzberg et al., 1987). Therefore, the imaging diagnosis must not be used as the primary diagnosis since this could lead to unnecessary surgical treatment.

In the study described here, arthroscopy was as effective as arthrography in diagnosing disk displacement. The arthroscopic diagnosis is a deduction, however, based on inference from associated pathological surface conditions, such as stretching of the posterior attachment, adhesions, and tears. This technique may be successful in the hands of the experienced diagnostician; however, TMJ arthroscopy is a relatively new procedure, and both normal and abnormal surface morphology and nomenclature are still being defined (Murakami and Hoshino, 1982). Liedberg and Westesson

(1986) found the diagnostic accuracy of upper compartment arthroscopy to be only 50 percent, with the error representing underdiagnosis of the disorder. The higher accuracy in the present study is probably due to the extent of the morphological changes present in the sample, unlimited observation time under experimental conditions, and the fact that the lower joint compartment was also examined in the cadaver material. Some apparent anterior displacement of the disk may also be a natural variation in location (Hellsing and Holmlund, 1985) or part of a natural adaptation process (see Chap. 10).

One of the most important pieces of diagnostic information and one of its diagnostic strengths, namely disk morphology, is commonly ignored in arthrography (see Chap. 10). Of course, this requires a double joint space procedure. Arthroscopy cannot provide this information since its use is restricted to the upper joint space at this time. CT and MRI, however, may produce similar disk morphology data to the double joint space arthrogram.

Future Directions for TMJ Imaging

As increasing numbers of TMJ arthroscopic procedures are performed, it is anticipated that the details of articular surface morphology will continue to be defined along with their clinical correlates (Murakami and Hoshino, 1985). At this time arthroscopy is the only technique reported to have therapeutic as well as diagnostic value (Murakami et al., 1986; Sanders, 1986).

A more widespread examination of diagnostic imaging is currently under way to include CT and MRI, and a larger sample should resolve some of the limitations of using autopsy material by including a wider range of ages and of joint morphology. The sample described earlier included only elderly individuals, and their joints displayed rather extensive morphologic changes. Without any information about the clinical status of these individuals before death, the clinical significance of the joint changes is unknown. Autopsy material taken from individuals who had a natural death provides a sample that on average is older than most of the patients in the TMJ clinics. The lack of material for dissection from a sample in a younger age range has prevented the important assessment of false-positive findings for imaging in the small sample studied to date. Nevertheless, with no useful animal model and limitations on comparative imaging in patients, cadavers remain our best source of information about anatomical relationships in the temporomandibular joint.

Summary

The choice of TMJ imaging technique should be based on the clinical diagnosis. Tomography is the technique of choice for imaging osseous changes. Double joint space arthrography in the tomographic mode is useful for examining articular disk morphology and position. Diagnostic arthroscopy reveals localized surface pathology in the upper joint space and contributes to a diagnosis of disk displacement by inference from associated disease.

References

Baldioceda F, Pullinger A, Bibb C: Distribution and histological character of condylar osseous defects. J Dent Res 66:319 (Abstr 1702), 1987.

Eckerdal O: Correlation between the tomographic image and the anatomy. Acta Radiol (Suppl 329): 52–73, 1973.

Hansson TL, Oberg T, Carlsson GE, Kopp S: Thickness of the soft tissue layers and the articular disc in the temporomandibular joint. Acta Odont Scand 35:77–83, 1977.

Hellsing G, Holmlund A: Development of anterior displacement in the temporomandibular joint: An autopsy study. J Pros Dent 53:397–401, 1985.

Helms CA, Richardson ML, Vogler JB, Hoddick WK: Computed tomography for diagnosing temporomandibular joint disk displacement. J Craniomandib Pract 3:24–26, 1984.

Katzberg RW, Westesson PL, Tallents RH, Sanchez-Woodworth RE, Svensson SA, Espeland MA: Comparison between magnetic resonance imaging and sagittal cryosectional anatomy of the normal temporomandibular joint. (Abst. 1844.) J Dent Res 66:337, 1987.

Kircos LT, Ortendahl DA, Arakawa M, Mark A: Demonstration of TMJ anterior disc position by MRI in asymptomatic subjects. (Abst. 1842.) J Dent Res 66:337, 1987.

Liedberg J, Westesson PL: Diagnostic accuracy of upper compartment arthroscopy of the temporomandibular joint: Correlation with postmortem morphology. Oral Surg 62:618–624, 1986.

Murakami K, Hoshino K: Regional anatomical nomenclature and arthroscopic terminology in human temporomandibular joints. Okajimas Folia Anat Jpn 58:745–760, 1982.

Murakami K, Hoshino K: Histological studies on the inner surfaces of the articular cavities of human temporomandibular joints with special reference to arthroscopic observations. Anat Anz Jena 160:167–177, 1985.

Murakami K, Matsuki M, Iizuka T, Ono T. Diagnostic arthroscopy of the TMJ: Differential diagnosis in patients with limited jaw opening. J Craniomandib Pract 4:118–126, 1986.

Pullinger A, Baldioceda F, Bibb C: Prediction of TMJ articular surface configuration from condylar osseous outline. (Abst. 1848.) J Dent Res 66:338, 1987.

Ross J: Arthrography of the TMJ, in Solberg WK, Clark GT (eds): Perspectives in Temporomandibular Disorders. Chicago, Quintessence, 1987, pp 69–88.

Sanders B: Arthroscopic surgery of the temporomandibular joint: Treatment of internal derangement with persistent closed lock. Oral Surg 62:361–372, 1986.

Solberg WK, Hansson TL, Nordstrom B: The temporomandibular joint in young adults at autopsy: A morphologic classification and evaluation. J Oral Rehab 12:303–321, 1985.

Westesson PL, Rohlin M: Internal derangement related to osteoarthrosis in temporomandibular joint autopsy specimens. Oral Surg Oral Med Oral Pathol 57:17–22, 1984.

10 Natural History and Pathologic Progression of Internal Derangements with Persistent Closed Lock /
Andrew G. Pullinger

This chapter reviews some of our understanding of the natural life history of TMJ internal derangements with particular reference to the outcome of disk displacement without reduction (closed lock). This information will be applied to generate an improved understanding of the goals of conservative and surgical treatment.

TMJ derangements are common in the general population (30 percent), although far fewer people complain of sufficient disability to seek treatment (Solberg et al., 1979; Pullinger and Monteiro, 1988). The appropriate questions are, "What factors predispose to or precipitate progression of these disorders to situations of pain, interference, and restriction, and what determines if the outcome is arthrotic breakdown or successful adaptation?"

Conservative versus Surgical Treatment Option

An adapted closed lock is not necessarily a serious problem and could be considered a successful response by the body to a difficult disk laxity problem so as to regain joint stability. Long-term outcome with simple conservative treatment in seven-year (Carlsson, 1985) and other follow-up studies (McNeill, 1985) indicates a recovery of range of jaw movement and few pain symptoms. Even the consequences of arthrosis with conservative therapies are generally favorable with few symptoms reported at seven-year follow-up, with crepitation being the predominant clinical sign (Rasmussen, 1981; Mejersjo, 1984). Crepitation per se is not a disabling condition. Thus Carlsson (1985) states that derangement and arthrosis should be considered benign disorders that respond well to conservative therapies.

Open TMJ surgical therapies have some favorable reports, especially for disk repair procedures (Benson and Keith, 1985; Dolwick et al., 1987). Finding suitable comparison populations and the methods of determining success, however, present significant problems in such studies. The long-term consequences of silicone and Teflon implant materials used in meniscectomy treatment of closed lock is under severe scrutiny because of the breakup of the materials (Ericksson and Westesson, 1986) and inflammatory reactions (El Deeb et al., 1987). In a 30-year follow-up of meniscectomy without implants, Eriksson and Westesson (1985) observed a normalized range of jaw opening and the absence of pain despite crepitation and notable radiographic changes. Experimental temporary placement of silicone implants induces a fibrous encapsulation that remains between the condyle and the fossa after the implant is removed (Barwick and Tucker, 1987) and might merit further research.

The American Association of Oral and Maxillofacial Surgeons (1984) recommends at least 35 mm of jaw opening for a postsurgical result to be described as successful. This is not particularly favorable considering the long-term recovery of range of motion in closed lock expected by more conservative therapy. Mejersjo and Carlsson (1983) followed a large group of TMJ patients treated by conservative methods. Of these, 20 percent complained of locking. After completion of active treatment, only 11 percent complained of locking, and at seven-year follow-up none complained of locking. Similarly, for the specific symptom of limited opening, in the total patient sample the figures were 35 percent, 13 percent, and 7 percent, respectively. Furthermore, caution should be expressed because sometimes TMJ symptoms are self-limiting. In a long-term follow-up of patients who had not responded during a course of conservative therapy, Greene and Laskin (1983) noted that half eventually became better regardless of whether they received more treatment. Similarly, 33 percent of another sample of TMJ patients who had elected not to proceed with treatment stated an excellent eventual outcome at follow-up (Clark et al., 1986). These last two studies did not differentiate locking.

At this time the only legitimate rationale for open TMJ surgery for closed lock may be intractable pain, and even then an adequate informed consent would have to include discussion of the above prognoses for the nonsurgical options (Rasmussen, 1981; Mejersjo and Carlsson, 1983; Mejersjo, 1984). The 1982 American Dental Association Conference on Temporomandibular Disorders recommends that TMJ surgery should be considered only for specific intracapsular pathology or for derangements if conservative treatments have failed.

Overall Treatment Goals

The appropriate treatment goals for temporomandibular disorders can be stated as follows: (1) symptomatic care; (2) achievement of an environment favorable for adaptation such that further breakdown is interrupted and the natural recovery time is reduced, both at an economical cost to the tissues.

TMJ Internal Derangements: Etiological Concepts

Functional Progression Theory

Disk displacement without reduction is most commonly explained as a functional progression (Dolwick et al., 1983) from disk-condyle incoordination (disk displacement with reduction, or clicking) to disk-condyle interference and restriction (disk displacement without reduction, or locking) with disk perforation and arthrosis stated as the eventual sequelae. This theory is built on cross-sectional information through TMJ arthrographic imaging of patients seeking treatment. Unfortunately, in the absence of longitudinal epidemiological studies, the risk factor for symptom progression for the general population is unknown. Magnetic resonance imaging (MRI), which avoids ionizing radiation, may hold promise for future population studies. From the epidemiology it is evident that most TMJ clicking does not progress to locking or even problem clicking. Although 30 to 50 percent of one population of young adults studied (Pullinger and Monteiro, 1988) reported an awareness of some TMJ clicking, only 5 to 8 percent complained of continual clicking and 4 to 7 percent that the clicking disturbed jaw function. The frequency of any locking, mostly momentary, was exceedingly low (less than 1 percent). It has been estimated that only 5 percent of the population will ever seek any TMJ treatment (Solberg et al., 1979). Nine percent of 70 TMJ patients with reciprocal clicking progressed to locking in a 3-year study (Lundh et al., 1987).

Rasmussen (1981) was able to classify the sequence of symptoms in subjects seeking treatment for TMJ arthropathy into six sequential phases (Table 10–1) using patient history and prospectively during treatment. These patients had presented with TMJ pain or restriction and radiographic condyle changes. Eighty percent of these patients reported at least one of the two phases of each of the clinical stages, and 50 percent reported all six phases. Nevertheless, the intermediate stage of arthropathy occurred without a preceding clicking or locking phase in 32 percent and 39 percent, respectively, which indicates that TMJ internal derangement is not the only route to TMJ arthrosis. Osteoarthrosis is the final outcome of many possible processes. Progression of closed lock to TMJ arthrosis would appear not to be inevitable (Pullinger and Seligman, 1987).

TABLE 10-1
Progression of Symptoms in TMJ Arthropathy Patients

STAGE	PHASE	MEDIAN DURATION (YR.)
Initial	1: Clicking	2.5
	2: Periodic locking	1.5
Intermediate	3: TMJ pain at rest	0.5
	4: TMJ pain on function	0.5
Terminal	5: Residual symptoms other than pain	2.25
	6: Absence of symptoms (Rasmussen, 1981)	2.3

Closed Lock of Sudden Onset

An absence of any history of TMJ clicking is not that unusual in closed lock patients. Typically, they may report awaking with severe jaw restriction as the first onset. In a retroactive review of 225 TMJ patients (Pullinger and Seligman, 1987), 18 percent (4/22) of patients with locking reported no prior history of TMJ derangement.

Pathophysiology of Disk Displacement Without Reduction

The explanations for both gradual or sudden symptom progression to closed lock are mostly speculative and probably involve several factors.

Sex Differences

Significantly more women than men have TMJ derangement symptoms (Solberg et al., 1979; Rieder et al., 1983) and possibly more serious or more progressive derangements (Pullinger and Monteiro, 1988). In a retrospective study of 225 TMJ patients (Pullinger and Seligman, 1987), all the patients with closed lock were women, compared to only 77 percent of those with disk displacement with reduction. Women also seem to have more TMJ surgeries for severe internal derangement problems as evidenced by the 40:1 female-to-male ratio described by McCoy and colleagues (1986).

Age

Interestingly, recent information indicates that the average age of patients with closed lock is younger than for those with disk displacement with reduction, 29.0 (S.D. 7.25 years) versus 34.6 (S.D. 11.1 years) (Pullinger and Seligman, 1987). This might indicate more than one pathophysiology or that the same factors have different outcomes when operating on different age groups: namely, that the consequence if experienced by younger women is more likely to be a more serious disk displacement without reduction. This is discussed further under "Laxity."

Trauma

Recent insight afforded by TMJ arthroscopy suggests a second hypothesis for the pathophysiology of derangements not based on direct traumatic stretching of ligaments and displacement of the disk. Synovitis with adhesion may be the main problem secondary to trauma, which then progressively interferes with smooth condylar translation, with subsequent articular connective tissue changes, disk distortion, and ligament elongation. The joint may adapt or become further restricted by adhesions or be destabilized by what then appears clinically to be a sudden disk displacement. Arthroscopy reveals that fibrillations and regions of localized synovitis can exist in the absence of clinical TMJ tenderness, which is an important consideration in the management of traumatic arthritis.

TMJ patients more frequently have a history of head or neck trauma and accidental or iatrogenic overmanipulation of the jaw compared to controls (Pullinger and Monteiro, in press). A history of trauma also differentiated symptomatic from asymptomatic controls with particular association to signs of TMJ clicking. It is apparent that men must better modulate and recover from the effects of direct and indirect jaw trauma. Although men presumably have greater exposure to jaw trauma through contact sports, it is rare to see a male patient with closed lock, and few present with problem reciprocal clicking requiring orthopedic therapy (condyle repositioning).

Nonspecified trauma was as much a factor in the history of patients with disk displacement with reduction, 63 percent, as with closed lock, 79 percent (Pullinger and Seligman, 1987). But surprisingly, disk displacement without reduction was more frequently associated with a history of the more major trauma of motor vehicle accidents, 71 percent, than was disk displacement with reduction, 45 percent. Such accidents frequently produce hyperpropulsion injuries to the jaw, which would correctly be termed "jaw lash," causing stretching of the diskal ligaments and partial disk displacement. Nevertheless, in this author's experience, this rarely seems to progress to a closed lock unless there is a preexisting disorder. Of closed lock cases involving major trauma, 36 percent proved to have histories of other preceding trauma (Pullinger and Seligman, unpublished).

Joint Laxity

Susceptibility to closed lock may be more associated with conditions of joint laxity. In the rheumatology literature, joint laxity is associated with younger age and with women (Scott et al., 1979) and predisposes to arthrosis in population studies. The greater angle of maximum jaw opening shown in young adult women in anthropometric studies (Pullinger et al., in press) does indicate a greater range of TM joint movement in women, which is probably an example of greater localized joint laxity. Results of studies attempting to associate generalized or benign hypermobility as an etiological factor in adult TMJ patients have been equivocal (Bates et al., 1984). In our own experience (Pullinger et al., in press), very few young adult men fulfill the 60 percent score criteria for generalized hypermobility, which therefore makes it unlikely that this is an important factor in men with TMJ derangements. Nevertheless, for both sexes, a situation of greater joint laxity may have existed around the time of initiation of many TMJ disorders that Egermark-Eriksson and coworkers (1981) show to be similar to adult prevalence, although not in severity, by the middle teenage years.

Temporomandibular Orthopedics

It is my interpretation that although a range of condyle position is found in normal functioning joints (Pullinger et al., 1985), the wider the interarticular space between the posterior slope of the articular eminence and the condyle, the greater inherent difficulty there is accommodating and preserving a biomechanically preferred biconcave disk shape in location. This then compromises optimal disc-condyle stability. Thus a posterior position of the condyle probably predisposes to disk instability, although other factors probably have to be operating for a displacement to occur.

A posterior condyle position has been described in 70 percent of both male and female TMJ patients with disk displacement (Pullinger et al., 1986) and as occurring in more female than male normals (Pullinger et al., 1985). The anterosuperior joint space visualized by computed tomographic imaging has been described as larger in joints with disk displacement (Christensen, in press). Most posterior condyle positions are probably innate and should not be explained as a condylar displacement, even though some superior adjustment of condyle position must occur (Hellsing et al., 1986).

Posterior condyle position and also inferior displacement of the condyle may deform or compromise the biomechanical function of the posterior band of the articular disk, permitting possible anterior displacement of the disk. In the experience of the UCLA Arthrographic Service (J. R. Ross, personal communication, 1986), it is not unusual in unilateral cases to discover the supposed asymptomatic condyle seated on the crest of the posterior band of the disk (Fig. 10–1). Such partial disk displacement may suddenly become an overt disk displacement with minimal apparent cause, such as a high filling, a hard bolus of food, or a minor trauma. In contrast, some authors relate minimal disk distortion in reducible disk displacements and report notable distortion in nonreducing closed locks, leading them to conclude that most disk distortion is secondary to the disk displacement rather than primary (Westesson et al., 1985). Hansson (1986), basing an opinion upon extensive work on condylar deviation in form, states the counterhypothesis: that disk displacement is a consequence of disk deformation and soft tissue changes in the joint components.

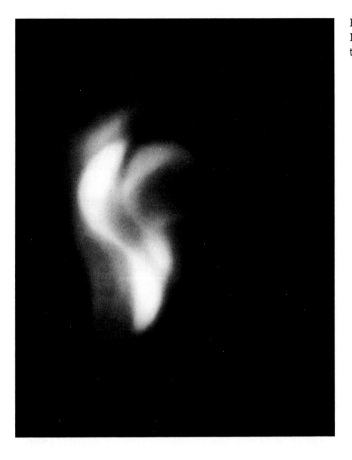

FIGURE 10–1 / TMJ arthrotomogram of disk and condyle in ICP. Note that the condyle is functioning on the posterior thickened part of the articular disk.

Dental Occlusion

Contrary to more traditional gnathologic beliefs, recent occlusion literature indicates that a small symmetrical slide between retruded condyle position and intercuspal position may afford some protection to the temporomandibular joint, whereas TMJ clicking more frequently accompanied a lack of occlusal slide (Pullinger et al., in press). In a sample of asymptomatic normals, there was no significant correlation between deep bite and the posterior position of the condyle (Pullinger et al., 1987b). That sample was too small to comment on Class II, division 2, as a specific subset. No difference existed, however, between any orthodontic class with respect to TMJ derangements in the epidemiological sample (Pullinger et al., in press). A weak relationship was shown between myalgia involving multiple sites and deep bite (Seligman et al., in press). Temporomandibular tenderness was more common in Class II, division 2, occlusions (Pullinger et al., in press).

Summary of Factors

In all probability no single factor is dominant and may only increase predisposition to TMJ derangement given the presence of coexisting factors or events.

Traditional statistical analyses of typical groups may be missing the problem because the biomechanics operating might be very individual-specific (Hannam, 1984). For example, by integrating mandibular kinematics and an MRI description of muscle angulations and mass together with occlusal variables, an improved understanding of the unique resolution of force vectors for each individual may be better obtained. This may unfortunately imply that deceptively similar occlusal states may generate very different loading effects and consequences.

Sequelae of Disk Displacement Without Reduction

Initial Phase

Despite initial painful restriction (Rasmussen, 1981), the longer outlook for a patient with closed lock is more hopeful with increased range of jaw movement and partial normalization by elongation of the posterior disk attachments, further disk deformation, and more disk displacement (Ericksson and Westesson, 1983). A continuous myospasm frequently occurs in the jaw elevator muscles during the early phases of locking and is likely to be the primary source of pain, rather than TMJ arthralgia. This is probably an example of muscle splinting provoked through an arthrokinetic reflex, which Isberg and colleagues (1985) described as caused by joint distraction as the condyle pathway becomes obstructed by the displacing articular disk in TMJ clicking.

Disk Deformation and Displacement

Westesson and coworkers (1985) concluded from arthrographic and anatomical study of autopsy material that disk displacement precedes disk deformation. Biconcave disk shapes were associated with disk displacement with reduction, and greater deformation and disk perforation with nonreducing disks. Deformation was rare in normal superiorly positioned disks. In cases with partial anterior displaced disks (displacement of only their lateral aspect), most disks preserved their biconcave shape in all other aspects except the region of displacement. Disk deformation was present in most cases of complete anterior displacement (mostly disk displacement without reduction). The latter group also contained most of the instances of disk perforation, predominantly in the posterior attachment. Other studies (see Chap. 9; Hanson and Oberg, 1977; Solberg et al., 1985) locate the area of greatest thinning or changes in the more lateral aspect of the disk. Westesson and Rohlin (1984) found partial anterior disk displacement in 22 percent of an autopsy sample, and 34 percent had complete anterior disk displacement. This is evidently higher than the 12 percent prevalence of disk displacement recorded by Hansson and coworkers (1983) in a young adult autopsy sample, which is a better match to the age of most TMJ patients attending clinics. An even higher frequency of disk displacement (100 percent) was seen in another older natural death autopsy group (see Chap. 9). It is feasible that some disk displacement occurs as a natural adjustment and adaptation so as to maintain TMJ stability with age. Hellsing and Holmlund (1985), on the other hand, explain some of the observed anterior disk position as a natural variation rather than as a displacement.

Interestingly, an absence of clicking in the arthrographic study by Eriksson and Westesson (1983) did not always imply normal disk function since 38 percent of joints with anterior disk displacement with reduction were silent. Reciprocal clicking in that same sample was considered a reliable sign of disk displacement with reduction. On the other hand, Macher and colleagues (1985) presented a case study of reciprocal clicking occurring with a nonreducing displaced disk in a case of osteoarthrosis; fibrous bands were suggested as responsible for the acoustic observations.

In the previous sample of disk displacement (Ericksson and Westesson, 1983) some sex differences were evident: nonreducing disk displacement was found in only 29 percent of men compared to 59 percent of women. Additionally, four women had reduced range of opening with a normal disk position; in retrospect this may have been a manifestation of adhesions.

In the opinion of Westesson and coworkers (1985), since disk deformation appears to be preceded by anterior disk displacement, early treatment of symptomatic derangements seems indicated.

Disk Elongation

Westesson and colleagues (1985) and Scapino (1983) have observed an increase in the length of the anterior recess in the lower joint compartment in joints with disk displacement. This is probably mostly indicative of elongation of the collateral discal ligaments. Normally the biconcave shape of the articular disk is biomehanically responsible for maintaining the disk-to-condyle position through all ranges of condyle translation. When the disk is displaced anteriorly, however, or the disk shape has become biplanar or biconvex, all the stabilizing function falls to the diskal ligaments. Elongation of the posterior ligaments and elastic tissue of the bilaminar zone inevitably occurs, which further compromises the retrusive return of the disk.

Figure 10–2 shows the degree of elongation possible. In this case of complete anterior disk displacement, probably at least 10 mm of ligament elongation has occurred plus extension of the anterior joint recess. The biconcave shape of the disk, however, is somewhat preserved.

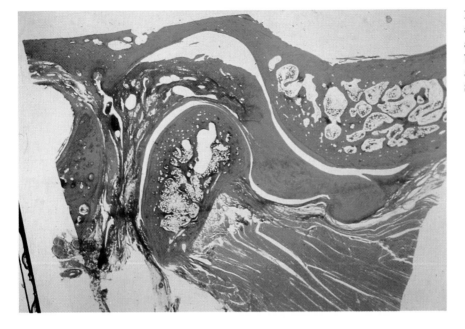

FIGURE 10–2 / Histological section of
a young adult with TMJ with complete
anterior disk displacement, showing
biconcave form and elongation of the
anterior recess. Courtesy of Dr. W.K.
Solberg.

Prognosis

In terms of prognosis, a partial anterior disk displacement (involving only the lateral aspect of the disk) would be easier to stabilize using a stabilization splint or condyle anterior repositioning and may even permit eventual return to the patient's original intercuspal position. A more complete anterior displacement would be more difficult to manipulate out of a closed lock, and if reduced would subsequently be more of a problem to stabilize to the condyle with repositioning, owing to the usually permanent diskal elongation and altered morphology. Most of such cases probably remain untreated or treated off the disk. Not enough is known of the healing potential of TMJ ligaments. On the other hand, the biconcave shape of the disk is preserved in this example (Fig. 10–2), which implies a biomechanically favorable shape to steady the disk if re-engagement between the condyle and the temporal bone were possible provided that no large translation movements occur in the earlier stage of treatment and there is no increase in joint space, such as in forceful jaw closure on a food bolus.

Figure 10–3 shows a severely displaced and distorted disk. Even if this could be unlocked by manipulation or disk surgery, there is little probability that the shape of the disk could be stabilized to the condyle. McCarty (1980) has stated that a dislocated disk that has undergone significant distortion cannot be reduced and stabilized to maintain a normal disk-condyle relationship. Furthermore, an extensive deviation in the form of the articular soft tissue is present on the superior aspect of the condyle shown in Figure 10–3, which would interfere with normal disk function. Current clinical radiographic examinations would not image this kind of soft tissue deformity, which may lead to a false-negative finding. Frequently the soft tissue contour cannot be predicted from the bone contour (Pullinger et al., 1987a).

Probably the most important requirement for a TMJ imaging technology for derangements is the ability to diagnose disk morphology since this may significantly affect treatment decisions and prognosis. The standard for disk imaging is still double-joint-space arthrography, but magnetic resonance holds considerable promise. Emphasis on diagnosis of disk displacement is probably overplayed since this information can usually be determined clinically and the vast majority of disk displacements are managed successfully without reduction of the disk. Loud clicking joints probably have retained some of their biconcave structure and may be more easily stabilized on the condyle. Softer clicks imply more disk flattening and will be more unstable until there has been sufficient flattening to permit noninterfering translation of the condyle.

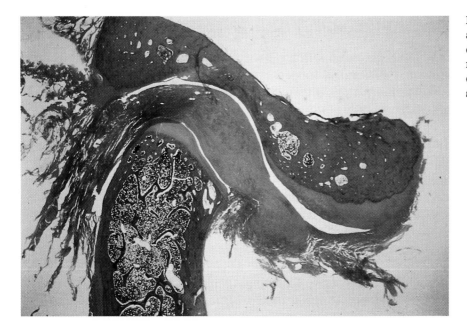

FIGURE 10–3 / Histological section of a young adult with TMJ with anterior disk displacement and distortion of disk morphology. Note the articular soft-tissue deviation in form on the condyle superiorly. Courtesy of Dr. W.K. Solberg.

TMJ Remodeling and Osteoarthrosis

In general, articular surface irregularities are more associated with deformed disks and more severe changes with completely anteriorly displaced disks (Ericksson and Westesson, 1983; Westesson and Rohlin, 1984), indicating that closed lock may be a precursor to osteoarthrosis in some cases (Westesson et al., 1985). Notwithstanding, caution should be employed before interpreting all subsequent radiographic changes as degenerative or arthrotic. Many radiographic changes would be more accurately described as adaptive remodeling. As stated earlier, recent histological studies showed that condyle osseous contours and osseous defects were not good predictors of the actual soft tissue articular surface (Pullinger et al., 1987a; Baldioceda et al., 1987).

Figure 10–4 shows that the articular soft tissue may biomechanically compensate for apparent osseous defects to maintain a smooth surface, at least in the short term. Conversely, clinical crepitation may not be a reliable sign of osteoarthrosis. Eriksson Westesson, and Rohlin (1985) were unable to find signs of osteoarthrosis in one-third of joints with crepitation operated on for disk displacement disorders. Hansson and coworkers (1983) associated most clinical crepitation with radiographic bone changes. Some of the differences in findings depend on the definition of arthrosis, which in the case of Eriksson and colleagues (1985) signified disk perforation and exposure of bone. Broader definitions of arthrosis which use remodeling of subchondral bone (Hansson, 1977) require caution to avoid overdiagnosis of radiographic changes. Clinical experience shows us that some closed locks adapt successfully without proceeding to degenerative joint disease even though signs of osseous remodeling may become evident.

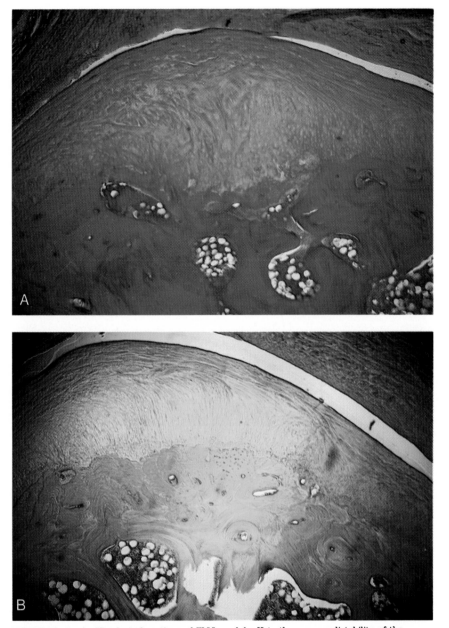

FIGURE 10–4 / Histological sections of TMJ condyle. Note the poor predictability of the actual soft-tissue articular surface and thickness based on the osseous contours of the condyle.

Remodeling Without Arthrosis

The mandibular condyle is capable of extensive remodeling without arthrosis, as seen in Figure 10–5. This shows a tomogram of a totally asymptomatic temporomandibular joint without any symptom history in either joint except for lighter ICP contacts on that side. In all probability this is an example of remodeling following an undiagnosed juvenile fracture. Since there are no signs of dysfunction, it is assumed that the articular tissues of the lining are intact.

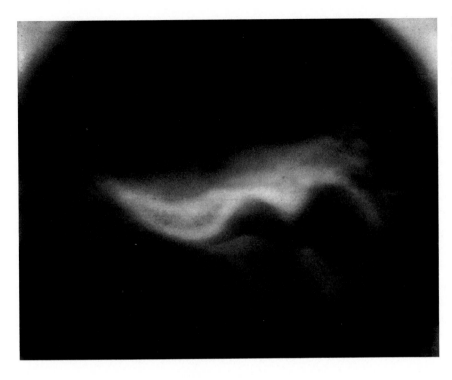

FIGURE 10-5 / TMJ tomogram
showing asymptomatic advanced
remodeling of the mandibular condyle.
Note the flattening and pointed
appearance of the condyle.

Adhesions

Some clinical crepitation probably signifies movement hesitation and areas of articular surface irregularity rather than arthrosis. The intra-articular adhesions visualized in diagnostic arthoscopy may contribute to such crepitation or may cause a suction cup or sticking effect on the disk.

Figure 10–6 of young adult TMJ autopsy material shows an extensive region of intra-articular adhesion as a continuous connective tissue incorporating the diskal tissue between the temporal bone and the condyle. This illustrates one important histological fact: that the normal lining connective tissue to the temporal bone and the condyle are the same tissue type as the articular disk. This adhesion would undoubtedly disturb condyle translation and also resist manipulation and distraction of the condyle for reduction of the disk. It is acknowledged that some of this appearance might be postmortem and artifactual change. Technically, it has proved exceptionally difficult to capture the more filamentous fibrillations (seen during joint hydration in arthroscopy) in histological sections since in situ these form a delicate three-dimensional web that is not represented in a single plane section.

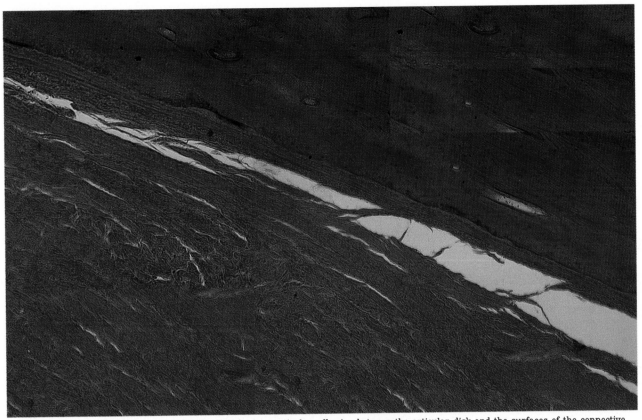

FIGURE 10–6 / Histological section of TMJ. Note the intraarticular adhesion between the articular disk and the surfaces of the connective tissue of the temporal bone.

Adaptation

The mandibular condyle has potential for adaptation. The layers of articular cartilage seem highly responsive to biomechanical changes to the TMJ during growth in experimental protrusive function studies (McNamara and Carlson, 1979). The mandibular condyle is capable of extensive remodeling without arthrosis as was seen in Figure 10–5. Although the tissue response to experimental protrusive function in young adult animals was similar to that during growth (McNamara et al., 1982), the adaptive capacity is considered more limited and highly variable. Because of the poorer adaptive capacity of adult joints, Hellsing and coworkers (1985) are rather skeptical about mandibular repositioning therapy in adults. They also present a case with surprising extensive remodeling, however, following repositioning treatment in which a double bony contour was generated in the posterior part of the condyle.

The altered biomechanics in TMJ internal derangements produces bony adaptation of the condyle and temporal bone in addition to soft tissue adaptation and postural adaptation of the mandible. To think of "disk recapturing" treatment in simple mechanical terms rather than as a complex biological adaptation is therefore an error that implies that neither the operator nor the patient is making an informed treatment decision. The factors determining whether the outcome is successful adaptation over time (Carlsson, 1985) or whether there will be disk and articular surface breakdown are not proven. Notwithstanding, the objective of any treatment is to promote any residual healing potential and to tilt the balance toward positive adaptation rather than tissue breakdown. This involves control of adverse loading, stabilizing the joint components, plus stabilizing the end point of mandibular closure. Most important, etiological factors must be addressed; to just address the derangement and ignore the etiological factors is to treat merely the effect of the problem and ignore the cause. This is probably one of the greatest causes of long-term failure of treatment for derangements.

Permanent morphological changes and reorientation of fibers have been described in displaced disks (Scapino, 1983). Figure 10–3 illustrates severe folding in the inferior surface of the disks at the presumed original seating location of the condyle. This condition would not have a favorable prognosis for disk repositioning. Hyperplastic change has been found in the bilaminar zone of a few patients with long-standing TMJ pain (Isberg et al., 1986). This has been attributed to continuing organization following a blood clot caused when a disk was severely displaced.

The displaced articular disk has some adaptive capacity and does not always progress to perforation and breakdown. As shown in Figure 10–7, the increased loading sustained by the anterior part of the bilaminar zone following dislocation of the disk may lead to fibrotic remodeling and extension of the disk posteriorly. Arterial changes and an increase in denser collagen have been noted in that location with a concomitant decrease in elastin (Scapino, 1983; Hall et al., 1984).

By definition, the repair response of the temporomandibular joint as a synovial joint is not mediated through vascular inflammation. Instead, the response of the articular surface is through resistive remodeling involving proliferation of the articular soft tissue layers. The more vascular bilaminar zone of the TMJ is unique, however, among synovial joints and holds definite potential for repair and metaplastic change. The inference from the elongation and flattening of the disk is an eventual reduction of disc-condyle interference and clicking. Also, as the anterior joint recess becomes elongated, the condyle will recover some translation movement along the inferior aspect of the disk. The implication is that such joints may become compound arthrodial joints in which translation movements occur in both joint compartments. This process evidently requires extensive histological change. Not much natural recovery of jaw opening is evident in a closed lock (apart from muscle splinting) in the first year of the problem. Attempts to stretch out the disk physically are too simplistic and have not been successful.

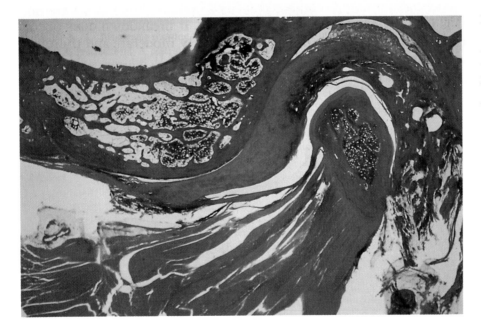

FIGURE 10–7 / Note the fibrotic (metaplastic) change occurring in the anterior part of the bilaminar zone in chronic disk displacement, resulting in posterior elongation of the fibrous disk rather than breakdown. Courtesy of Dr. W.K. Solberg.